A GUIDE TO THE NURSING OF THE AGING

Clinical Nursing Diagnosis Series

A GUIDE TO THE NURSING OF THE AGING

Charlotte Eliopoulos, RN, MPH

Consultant, Baltimore, Maryland

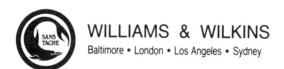

WILLIAMS & WILKINS
Baltimore • London • Los Angeles • Sydney

Editor: Mary Paquette
Associate Editor: Linda Napora
Copy Editor: Catherine Chambers
Design: A. Marshall Licht
Illustration Planning: Lorraine Wrzosek
Production: Anne Seitz

Accurate indications, adverse reactions, and dosage schedules for drugs are
provided in this book, but it is possible that they may change. The reader
is urged to review the package information data of the manufacturers of
the medications mentioned.

Printed in the United States of America

Library of Congress Cataloging in Publication Data
Eliopoulos, Charlotte.
  A guide to the nursing of the aging.

  (Clinical nursing diagnosis series)
  Includes index.
  1. Geriatric nursing. I. Title. II. Series.
[DNLM: 1. Geriatric Nursing. WY 152 E42ga]
RC954.E45 1987   610.73′65   87-8116
ISBN 0-683-09562-5

87 88 89 90   10 9 8 7 6 5 4 3 2 1

PREFACE

Although the specialty of gerontologic nursing is relatively new, nursing's history of caring for the elderly is not. Long before it became popular or profitable for other professionals to become involved with older adults, nurses assumed major responsibility for staffing institutions, taking services into the elderly's homes, and using their own homes to provide room, board, and personal care to the elderly as a forerunner to today's nursing home.

It was not until the 1960s that the unique aspects of nursing the aged were acknowledged to any significant degree. In 1961 the American Nurses' Association recommended the development of a special interest group for geriatric nurses, leading to the first national meeting of the Conference Group on Geriatric Nursing Practice the following year. In 1966 the ANA launched the Division of Geriatric Nursing. Within the decade that followed significant strides were made: Standards for Geriatric Nursing Practice emerged, certification in the specialty developed, literature in the field increased more than tenfold, and the Division changed its name from Geriatric to Gerontological Nursing to reflect the broader scope of nursing's role with aging persons. The growth in the quality and quantity of gerontologic practitioners and the sophistication and professionalization of the specialty have been steady since that time. Today, the specialty of nursing the aged is receiving the credibility and respect it deserves.

The development of nursing diagnoses has followed a path similar to that of the specialty of gerontologic nursing. Nursing historically had contributed uniquely to patient care but failed to describe that contribution in a manner that helped to differentiate it from medical practice. Through the 1960s and 1970s nurse theorists attempted to design nursing models, such as Ray's Adaptation Model, Orem's Self-Care Theory, and Roger's Life Processes. These nursing theories received lukewarm reception by many nurses who viewed them as too academic or irrelevant to their practice. Then came nursing diagnosis! When the National Group for the Classification of Nursing Diagnosis held its first meeting in 1973 there were those skeptics ready to judge nursing diagnosis as another academic exercise; but the momentum grew, as did the number of nurses who saw the relevancy of nursing diagnosis to their practices. Nursing diagnosis made logical sense and meshed nicely into the nursing process that most nurses understood.

It is interesting that the advancement of gerontologic nursing and nursing diagnosis occurred within similar time frames, although down separate paths, because when the major problems of the geriatric client are considered it is easy to see that they fall within the realm of nursing to diagnose and treat. Ask nurses who work with the elderly what problems consume their time and efforts and it will not be diabetes, congestive heart failure, cancer, or other medical diagnoses but the nursing diagnoses generated from them, such as potential for injury, noncompliance, knowledge deficit, impaired physical mobility, and self-care deficit. Thus, the marriage of geriatric nursing and nursing diagnosis seems appropriate and natural.

The purpose of this book is to present major geriatric nursing problems within a nursing diagnosis framework. Practical information is presented in an easily retrievable format to offer guidance to nurses who wish to implement this framework into their practice. For the new user of nursing diagnosis, time and practice in using this approach may be required to gain comfort and skill in its use. However, once nurses incorporate nursing diagnosis into their practices they will discover that it contributes to more organized care delivery, the demonstration of nursing's unique practice realm, and a foundation for research and knowledge development.

Special appreciation is expressed to Mary Paquette for her invaluable editorial assistance. Through frustrating and confounding times in this book's development she consistently provided the guidance and patience vital to keeping the momentum going.

Charlotte Eliopoulos

CONTENTS

TABLES

INTRODUCTION

A Guide to the Nursing of the Aging is one of the first clinical practice books to be organized strictly around a nursing model rather than around a medical model.

Nurses do not plan and implement their care based on medical diagnoses per se; they provide care for the patient's problems and concerns that are a result of the medical diagnoses. Many of these problems and concerns—now classified as nursing diagnoses—occur again and again with different medical diagnoses (e.g., fluid balance, nutritional alterations, grieving). Consequently, they generate some basic or generic processes. These generic nursing processes are modified, of course, by the impact of a specific medical diagnosis on the individual. *A Guide to the Nursing of the Aging* presents its content in precisely this way. A basic or generic nursing care plan is presented for a given nursing diagnosis followed by supplemental care for a selected medical diagnosis.

This book utilizes Gordon's functional health patterns (FHP) and nursing diagnosis. The nursing diagnosis statements are generally from the list approved by the North American Nursing Diagnosis Association (NANDA). Each functional health pattern is a separate chapter, and nursing diagnoses that may fall within that specific pattern are included in the chapter. Not every functional health pattern or every nursing diagnosis is included; only those that relate to the most common concerns in the nursing of the aged.

There is an implicit conceptual model of nursing and manner of application of the nursing process associated with the NANDA list. There is room for concept-overlap in this taxonomy. For example, the nursing diagnosis "anxiety" may be closely related to another one such as "ineffective airway clearance" or "ineffective family coping." Thus, one health problem may have several related nursing diagnoses. The reader is urged to look under several applicable diagnoses for related information.

In this book, the medical diagnoses appear as selected health problems frequently associated with a particular nursing diagnosis and are under the nursing diagnoses that have the most significant impact, and vice versa. Thus, if you want information about caring for an older adult with angina pectoris, you will not find it under the cardiovascular system; you will find it under the nursing diagnosis "Alteration in Tissue Perfusion: Cardiac."

A look at chapter 7, *Activity-Exercise Functional Health Pattern*, will be illustrative. The chapter opens with general information on activity and exercise, how these concepts apply to the elderly, and some of the medical problems that affect activity and exercise. Next, the author addresses the nursing diagnosis of "Alteration in Cardiac Output: Decreased" via a generic (basic) care plan. When using the generic nursing care plan, the nurse must use judgment to select the specific assessments, interventions, and evaluations that pertain to the specific older adult for whom the care is planned. The growth and development, medical diagnosis, abilities, knowledge, and motivation of patient and family may all affect the specific plan of care. Selected health problems that impact significantly on this nursing diagnosis (e.g., myocardial infarction) are then presented along with additional nursing care necessitated by this particular medical diagnosis. The reader is also referred to alternate or additional nursing diagnoses necessary to complete the plan of care.

Organizing nursing facts and content in this unique way is an ongoing challenge for all concerned. *A Guide to the Nursing of the Aging* is the second volume in the Clinical Nursing Diagnosis Series.

SECTION I

GENERAL CONSIDERATIONS

CHAPTER 1

NURSING AND THE AGING

Geriatrics, Gerontology, and Nursing

Historically there always has been interest in the elderly and the aging process. As early as the 6th century BC, Taoism promoted old age as the epitome of life and a reflection of a tremendous accomplishment. During the 5th century BC, Confucius proposed that the greater one's age, the greater the honor and respect entitled. In the centuries that followed, diverse reactions to old age and aging emerged. The early Egyptians invested considerable effort in seeking eternal youth. Plato advocated elders as society's leaders and recommended techniques for healthy aging, while Aristotle wished to exclude the elderly from important societal matters. Throughout the Dark Ages and Middle Ages the elderly held a low status and lead difficult existences. It primarily has been in this century that the increased numbers of old people and greater sensitivity to all human beings have caused the elderly to gain a new, positive recognition and enjoy a better life.

Geriatrics vs. Gerontology

The terms *geriatrics* and *gerontology* often are used interchangeably although there is a difference in their meanings.

Geriatrics is the branch of medicine concerned with the illnesses of old age and their care. Gerontology is the scientific study of the factors impacting the normal aging process and the effects of aging. In a true sense they are not synonymous.

Much of the past interest in gerontology revolved around interests in achieving immortality and eternal youth, witnessed by various potions and fountains of youth that were promoted at different times. It has only been

3

in the last century that increasingly sophisticated research interest has developed in learning about normal aging so that individuals could understand how to age in a healthy manner. Findings such as the correlation of parents' longevity to their offspring's longevity, and the importance of proper nutrition, exercise, rest, and stress management to healthy aging have been some of the outcomes of gerontologic research.

Nascher wrote the first geriatric textbook in 1914, but only in recent years has a tremendous growth in gerontology been noted. In the past, many pathologies (such as confusion, incontinence, and immobility) were accepted as expected outcomes of growing old. Unique norms in vital signs and laboratory findings were not known and the elderly were given unnecessary treatments to achieve norms for younger aged persons. Fortunately, research findings have given insight into normality and pathology in late life, and appropriate, age-specific care measures have been, and are still being, developed.

One of the exciting aspects of these specialties is that they are young and rapidly developing. Professionals in this area are afforded an opportunity seldom available in other fields, the chance to influence the development of a specialty.

Nursing

Long before it became a popular specialty, the care of the elderly was a responsibility and interest of nursing. Nurses have traditionally cared for the ill aged in hospitals, nursing homes, alms houses, retirement centers, and at home. In fact, the term "nursing home" stemmed from room-and-board houses operated by nurses or women who called themselves nurses. Geriatric nursing, because of the low status and salaries offered, was not a practice area that drew a great number of highly prepared or competent nurses. Often the nurses drawn to geriatric care were those who could not function well in other settings; thus, the stigma associated with this specialty was perpetuated. It wasn't until the early 1960s that a specialty group for geriatric nurses was promoted by the American Nurses' Association. Clinical research, teaching, and administrative leadership in this specialty has developed significantly as growing numbers of well-prepared, dynamic nurses are learning the challenges of working with the elderly. The years that followed brought significant growth for the specialty.

1966   Geriatric Nursing Division of ANA developed.
1969   Standards for Geriatric Nursing Practice written.
1975   Certification in Geriatric Nursing offered; first journal dedicated to specialty, *Journal of Gerontological Nursing*, published.

In 1976, when the ANA changed the specialty division from Geriatric Nursing to Gerontological Nursing, more than a name change occurred. A recognition of nurses' broad involvement with all aging persons was acknowledged. Whereas geriatric nursing focuses on the care of ill older people, gerontologic nursing includes health maintenance, illness prevention, illness management, and quality of life promotion. The scope of the gerontologic nurse is greater.

Who Are Gerontologic Nurses?

Only a small fraction of registered nurses, 7.7%, are employed in geriatric facilities. Although these nurses are often thought to be the primary ger ontologic nursing providers, there are nurses providing significant services to the elderly in a variety of other settings, including

- acute hospitals: many hospitals are discovering that a majority of their medical-surgical beds are filled by persons over age 65. Hospital clinics have replaced the community general practitioner as the source of medical care, so increasing numbers of elderly are served by outpatient departments.
- home health agencies: the largest portion of home health agencies' caseloads are older adults. Reimbursement policies that discourage in-patient care have resulted in greater numbers of elderly being seen with serious chronic diseases.
- rehabilitation centers: the realization that an improved functional status will add quality years to an impaired older person's life, and be cost effective, has launched geriatric rehabilitation as an increasingly grow-ing specialty.
- mental health centers: depressions and dementias are major problems affecting the older population and recent advancements in problem identification and therapeutic approaches have increased the elderly's use of outpatient psychiatric services to address these and other prob-lems.
- day treatment, day care: a variety of community-based programs have been developed as alternatives to institutionalization.
- sheltered housing, life care, retirement centers: new forms of health services are emerging in response to the changing needs and life-styles of new generations of older adults.

Even if nurses are in specialties catering to younger individuals, such as maternal and child health, they may still confront geriatric care issues as they work with families who have aged relatives. Thus, it is the rare nurse who is not affected by or able to impact geriatric care issues.

Roles of Gerontologic Nurses

One of the exciting aspects of gerontologic nursing is the ability to utilize a wide range of knowledge and skill in delivering services, such as medical-surgical, psychiatric, and community nursing; pharmacology; nutrition; than-atology; sociology; and psychology. This background is necessary to fulfill the diverse roles in gerontologic nursing.

Teacher.   Healthy aging starts early in life and so does education on prac-tices to facilitate this process. The gerontologic nurse teaches persons of all ages the principles of good hygiene, nutrition, exercises, rest, stress manage-ment, and prevention of illness and injury. With the high prevalence of chronic illness among the elderly, nurses also instruct in management of the condition, including special diets, safe medication use, and treatment techniques.

Counselor.   Aging persons and their families face issues and decisions for which they have had little preparation, such as retirement, finding a nursing home, caring for a sick spouse at home, losing a spouse, and grandparenting. The nurse can serve as a catalyst in helping individuals manage these situations by providing information, raising issues for consideration, guiding discussions, and linking with resources. In this way the nurse is strengthening individuals' abilities to deal with problems independently.

Agent.   There are many times when people cannot do for themselves and require nursing services to partially or totally assist them. "Doing for" older persons is not always necessary and often is not therapeutic. When an illness or handicap exists and persons are unable to care for themselves independently, nurses need to first evaluate the barriers to self-care, which could include the lack of knowledge or skills in care techniques; physical, emotional, or socioeconomic limitations; beliefs and attitudes; environmental obstacles; or motivation. Nursing actions should address the elimination or minimization of those barriers. Only when people are truly incapable of self-care (e.g., unconscious, confused, in need of a special treatment) should nurses assume the function of completing actions for individuals.

Advocate.   Advocacy takes many forms in gerontologic nursing. For the individual patient the nurse must ensure that the patient's personal preferences and needs are respected, and that the patient is able to play an active role in decision making and the care process. For the elderly, as a group, the nurse can support and recommend policies and programs that address needs in a humane and practical way. This may be particularly important now to balance cost-saving measures against service need and quality. For the specialty the nurse needs to promote the status and practice of gerontologic nursing.

Specific situations may find nurses filling additional roles, such as administrator, manager, consultant, and practitioner. Regardless of the position held, the gerontologic nurse's ultimate goal is to promote the highest level of health, function, and well-being in aging persons.

The challenges for gerontologic nurses in the future will be to continue the advancement of the specialty, prepare and recruit more nurses into this practice area, discover and implement new knowledge and skills, and improve the competency of all care givers working with the elderly.

The Nursing Process and the Elderly

Many of the needs presented by the aged can be appropriately identified and managed by nurses. The fact that nursing personnel are the major source of manpower in geriatric care attests to the significant role of nursing. Professional nursing meets this challenge by offering services in a planned, organized, and individualized manner rather than approaching care needs in a fragmented manner or solely through the fulfillment of medical orders. This systematic approach to nursing care is called the nursing process and consists of four general components: assessment, diagnosis and planning, implementation, and evaluation.

Assessment.   Assessment is the process of collecting and analyzing data. It is an ongoing activity and not a one-time snapshot of the patient. Table 1.1 outlines some of the data reviewed during the assessment and possible findings in older persons.

The quality and quantity of data collected can depend upon the patient's level of comfort during the assessment. Rapport must be established as a first step. Many elderly have had little experience being interviewed and may be less open than today's younger generations in discussing their bodily func-

Table 1.1   Assessment Categories and Possible Findings in the Older Adult

Data	Possible Findings
Name, date of birth	Language barriers Memory deficits
Address, telephone	Inadequate housing Multigenerational household (support system, problems) Social isolation
Religion	Dietary and other practices Services provided
Education	Illiteracy Inability to understand directions Interests, leisure activities
Contact person	Absence of support system Family relationships
Employment status	Financial problems Poor adjustment to retirement Occupational-related illness Unique skills, interests Self-concept disturbances
Financial status	Expenses exceed income Insufficient money to comply with health management needs Feelings of insecurity Not receiving benefits to which entitled
Family profile	No family resources Key figures in patient's life Support systems Ineffective relationships Ineffective coping patterns Family-imposed burdens Adjustment to widowhood, role changes
Life-style/social activities	Inability to maintain home Overwhelming responsibilities Fears Participation in family activities Recent changes

(continued)

Table 1.1   Assessment Categories and Possible Findings in the Older Adult (continued)

Data	Possible Findings
	Activity level alterations Role of pets Inadequate transportation Poor self-concept
Typical day	Activity intolerance Alterations in functions, responsibilities Rest and sleep disturbances Uneven distribution of activities
Activities of daily living	Deficits Alterations Compensatory mechanisms Use of assistive devices
Self-appraisal of health	Unrealistic views Denial Knowledge deficit Noncompliance
Health practices	Indulgence in foods Medication, alcohol abuse Unconventional practices
Health goal	Denial Unrealistic understanding Poor self-concept
Medication profile	Abuse Allergies Knowledge deficit Self-diagnosis and prescription Under- or over-medication
Body temperature	Subnormal Febrile
Pulse	Irregularities
Blood pressure	Hypo- or hypertension Postural changes
Respirations	Weak, shallow Ineffective gas exchange Shortness of breath
Height	Age-related reduction Reduction associated with spinal curvature, flexion contractures
Weight	Malnutrition Disease-related loss or gain
Skin condition	Poor turgor Rashes Ulcers, wounds Bruises Signs of abuse Poor hygienic practices
Mobility status	Gait disturbances Inability to climb stairs, transfer Contractures

Table 1.1 Assessment Categories and Possible Findings in the Older Adult (continued)

Data	Possible Findings
	Pain
	Need for assistance, assistive device
Dental status	Edentulous
	Halitosis
	Poorly fitting dentures
	Gum disease
Eating pattern	Inadequate or excessive food intake
	Likes and dislikes
	Anorexia
	Allergies
	Unique cultural, religious practices
	Digestion problems
	Food restrictions
	Amount of fluid intake
Elimination pattern	Urinary frequency, urgency
	Incontinence
	Constipation
	Bowel regularity
	Laxative abuse
	Self-imposed fluid restrictions
	Hemorrhoidal pain
Hearing ability	Conductive loss
	Perceptive loss
	Cerumen impaction
	Dependence on lip reading
Visual ability	Presbyopia
	Decreased peripheral vision
	Poor color discrimination
	Inadequate corrective lenses
	Cataracts
Tactile sensations	Inability to discriminate temperatures, textures, pressure
	Altered pain sensation
Sleep pattern	Alterations due to physical or mental illness
	Interruptions
	Medication abuse, reactions
	Insufficient activity
Sexual history	Impotence
	Poor self-concept
	Misinformation
	Lack of opportunity
	Guilt
	Discomfort, dysphoria
Mental status	Disorientation, confusion
	Flat affect
	Memory deficits
	Personality changes
	Poor judgment
	Medication reactions
	Undiagnosed physical problem

(continued)

Table 1.1   Assessment Categories and Possible Findings in the Older Adult (continued)

Data	Possible Findings
Medical diagnoses	Knowledge deficits Ineffective coping Self-care deficits Denial Need for assistance, assistive devices Noncompliance with treatment plan

tions, social problems, and feelings. They need to understand how this information will benefit their care and that it will be respected and held in confidence. Patients should know that they can feel free to ask questions or for clarification of words they do not understand. It should be remembered that more time may be needed to assess older persons to allow for slower responses and the review of the longer life history they possess. Memory may be poor and special hints to trigger recall are needed. Instead of asking if they have any allergies, it may be more fruitful to ask if they have ever become sick or developed a rash from eggs, tomatoes, any other food, drugs, lotions, materials, etc. Since interviews can be stressful events for older persons, memory can be further handicapped. Sensitivity is needed as the elderly have difficulty recalling information they should know. It may be useful to avoid dwelling on unanswered questions and return to them at a later time. Be sure to avoid jargon that patients may not understand and compensate for sensory deficits that could interfere with effective communication.

Environmental factors can affect the assessment positively and negatively. The area used should afford privacy and not be in the midst of noise and traffic that could act as detractors. The sensitivity of older persons to lower temperatures could reduce their ability to be attentive and comfortable if the room is too cool. A temperature of 75°F (24°C) is usually adequate; but confirm this with the patient. Seat the patient approximately 4 feet in front of the nurse to assure maximum visibility and allow for an adequate social distance. Control the room for glare (fluorescent lighting, direct sunlight through windows) that will be more bothersome to older eyes. Have bathroom facilities nearby and inform the patient of their location. Ensure that the seating offers comfort and support: it can be quite difficult for an older person to spend an hour lying on a hard examining table or sitting on a stool.

All senses are used in performing an assessment. General appearance, grooming and hygienic practices, appropriateness and style of clothing, posture and limitations in function can be observed; through physical examination more data can be derived. The nurse's ears can detect problems such as the clicking of poorly fitting dentures, wheezes, coughs, and unusual voice quality. Odors can reflect poor hygienic practices, incontinence, discharge, infectious processes, alcohol use, acidosis, or liver disease. The decreased olfaction of the elderly may cause them to be unaware of such odors on themselves. By touch the nurse can determine skin temperature, turgor, painful sites, and the patient's reactions to physical contact from others.

Inspection, auscultation, palpation, and percussion skills can be utilized in the assessment. Texts on physical assessment can assist the nurse in gaining more depth into these areas of examination.

Nursing Diagnosis and Planning. The wealth of history and problems older people possess demand that data collected be organized and prioritized so that appropriate care can be planned. Data should be analyzed for existing and potential problems. From these problems nursing diagnoses can be formulated (Table 1.2). A nursing diagnosis is a statement of a problem that nurses have the knowledge, skills and legal authority to assess and manage. In that respect it differs from a medical diagnosis, for example:

Medical diagnosis	*Nursing diagnosis*
Arthritis	Alteration in comfort: pain
	Impaired physical mobility
Paranoia	Impaired social interactions
	Alteration in thought processes

Thus, the nurse defines the problem in a manner that can be diagnosed and treated within the realm of nursing.

A nursing diagnosis is a two-part statement: the problem, sign, or symptom (diagnosis) and the cause or contributing factor. These components are linked by the phrase *related to*. The diagnosis presented in Table 1.2 are those that have been accepted for nursing practice and form a standardized list from which diagnoses can be selected. The contributing or causative factors

Table 1.2 Accepted Nursing Diagnoses (NANDA 1986)

Activity intolerance
Adjustment, impaired
Airway clearance, ineffective
Anxiety: mild, moderate, severe, panic
Body temperature, alteration in: potential
Bowel elimination, alteration in: constipation
Bowel elimination, alteration in: diarrhea
Bowel elimination, alteration in: incontinence
Breathing pattern, ineffective
Cardiac output, alteration in: decreased
Comfort, alteration in: pain
Comfort, alteration in: chronic pain
Communication, impaired: verbal
Coping, family: potential for growth
Coping, ineffective family: compromised
Coping, ineffective family: disabling
Coping, ineffective individual
Diversional activity deficit
Family process, alteration in
Fear
Fluid volume, alteration in: excess
Fluid volume deficit
Gas exchange, impaired

(continued)

Table 1.2   Accepted Nursing Diagnoses (continued)

Grieving, anticipatory
Grieving, dysfunctional
Growth and development, alteration in
Health maintenance, alteration in
Home maintenance management, impaired
Hyperthermia
Hypothermia
Incontinence, functional
Incontinence, reflex
Incontinence, stress
Incontinence, total
Incontinence, urge
Infection, potential for
Injury, potential for: poisoning, suffocation, trauma
Knowledge deficit (specify)
Mobility, impaired physical
Noncompliance (specify)
Nutrition, alteration in: less than body requirements
Nutrition, alteration in: more than body requirements
Oral mucous membrane, alteration in
Parenting, alteration in
Post trauma response
Powerlessness
Rape trauma syndrome
Self-care deficit: feeding, bathing/hygiene, dressing/grooming, toileting
Self-concept, disturbance in: body image, self-esteem, role performance, personal
   identity
Sensory-perceptual alteration: visual, auditory, kinesthetic, gustatory, tactile, olfactory
Sexual dysfunction
Sexuality patterns, alteration in
Skin integrity, impairment of
Sleep pattern disturbance
Social interaction, impaired
Social isolation
Spiritual distress (distress of the human spirit)
Swallowing, impaired
Thermoregulation, ineffective
Thought processes, alteration in
Tissue integrity, impaired
Tissue perfusion, alteration in: cerebral, cardiopulmonary, renal, gastrointestinal,
   peripheral
Unilateral neglect
Urinary elimination, alteration in patterns
Urinary retention
Violence, potential for: self-directed or directed at others

can be numerous and diverse and rest on the nurse's assessment findings from the individual patient. For example

- Activity intolerance related to stiff joints and pain
- Activity intolerance related to depressed state
- Fluid volume deficit related to cognitive inability to drink
- Fluid volume deficit related to diarrhea
- Self-care deficit: toileting related to immobility from fracture
- Self-care deficit: toileting related to cognitive inability to recognize need
  to void

In each of the above pairs it can be seen that the contributing/causative factor is important to distinguish because interventions will differ significantly with each reason behind the diagnosis. Once the diagnostic statement is made, care can be planned accordingly. Table 1.3 gives examples of potential risks for the older patient and possible related nursing diagnoses. The goal of the nursing care and outcome criteria for the patient are established at this time.

Table 1.3 Nursing Diagnoses for the Older Patient

Potential Risks Resulting from Age-related Changes	Related Nursing Diagnoses
Memory deficits	Alteration in health maintenance Noncompliance Potential for injury Impaired home maintenance management Knowledge deficit Anxiety Disturbance in self-concept Impaired social interactions
Slower learning of new information	Alteration in health maintenance Noncompliance Knowledge deficit Anxiety
Being stereotyped	Anxiety Powerlessness Disturbance in self-concept Alteration in family process Impaired social interactions
Dehydration	Fluid volume deficit Impairment of skin integrity Alteration in oral mucous membrane Alteration in bowel elimination: constipation Alteration in patterns of urinary elimination
Hypothermia	Potential alteration in body temperature Ineffective thermal regulation
Infection	Alteration in health maintenance Alteration in nutrition: less than body requirements Impairment of skin integrity Activity intolerance Sleep pattern disturbance Alteration in comfort: pain Social isolation
Poor circulation	Potential for infection Impairment of skin integrity Activity intolerance Alteration in tissue perfusion
Reduced gas exchange	Potential for infection Activity intolerance Ineffective airway clearance Ineffective breathing patterns Impaired gas exchange Alteration in thought processes
Aspiration	Potential for infection Ineffective airway clearance

(continued)

Table 1.3   Nursing Diagnoses for the Older Patient (continued)

Potential Risks Resulting from Age-related Changes	Related Nursing Diagnoses
	Impaired gas exchange Alteration in comfort: pain Anxiety Fear
Anorexia	Fluid volume deficit Potential for infection Alteration in nutrition: less than body requirements Alteration in bowel elimination: constipation Alteration in thought processes
Indigestion	Alteration in nutrition: less than body requirements Alteration in comfort: pain
Constipation	Alteration in nutrition: less than body requirements Alteration in bowel elimination: constipation Alteration in comfort: pain
Malabsorption of nutrients	Potential for infection Alteration in nutrition: less than body requirements Activity intolerance Impaired physical activity
Delayed absorption, metabolism and excretion of drugs	Potential for injury Self-care deficit Knowledge deficit Alteration in thought processes
Urinary frequency and urgency	Potential for injury Fluid volume deficit Impairment of skin integrity Alteration in patterns of urinary elimination Sleep pattern disturbance Anxiety Disturbance in self-concept Social isolation Reflex incontinence
Stress incontinence	Functional incontinence Potential for injury Impairment of skin integrity Alteration in patterns of urinary elimination Diversional activity deficit Anxiety Disturbance in self-concept Social isolation
Prostatic hypertrophy	Potential for infection Alteration in patterns of urinary elimination Sleep pattern disturbance Anxiety Disturbance in self-concept Altered sexuality patterns
Senile vaginitis	Impairment of skin integrity Alteration in comfort: pain Altered sexuality patterns
Dyspareunia	Alteration in comfort: pain Anxiety

Table 1.3   Nursing Diagnoses for the Older Patient (continued)

Potential Risks Resulting from Age-related Changes	Related Nursing Diagnoses
	Disturbance in self-concept
	Sexual dysfunction
Fractures	Alteration in health maintenance
	Potential for injury
	Impairment of skin integrity
	Activity intolerance
	Diversional activity deficit
	Impaired home maintenance management
	Impaired physical mobility
	Self-care deficit
	Alteration in comfort: pain
	Anxiety
	Powerlessness
	Disturbance in self-concept
	Sexual dysfunction
Immobility; range of motion	Alteration in health maintenance
	Potential for injury
	Potential for infection
	Impairment of skin integrity
	Alteration in bowel elimination: constipation
	Activity intolerance
	Ineffective breathing patterns
	Diversional activity deficit
	Impaired home maintenance management
	Impaired physical mobility
	Self-care deficit
	Powerlessness
	Disturbance in self-concept
	Social isolation
Muscle tremors and cramps	Activity intolerance
	Impaired physical mobility
	Sleep pattern disturbance
	Alteration in comfort: pain
Skin breakdown	Potential for infection
	Impairment of skin integrity
	Alteration in comfort: pain
	Disturbance in self-concept

Implementation.   Perhaps the strongest area of nursing practice has been implementation, because traditionally nurses have been taught the procedures involved in delivering care, however, this phase of the nursing process can only be as strong as the phases preceding it. Nursing actions should support the plan of care established. It must be remembered that with older patients

- more time may be required in delivering care due to age-related changes
- consistency of techniques and care givers can aid in minimizing stress
- needs change and must be reassessed continuously
- multidisciplinary care is often required and beneficial

- promoting their self-care ability or increasing the skills of family care givers can increase independence and feelings of normality.

Evaluation. Evaluation is an on-going and "fine tuning" phase in which necessary adjustments to care are detected and made. Evaluation can be done informally during care activities or formally through audits. Nurses must not only consider if the desired results were achieved, but if they were achieved most effectively and efficiently for the patient and the family unit. For example, hourly reality orientation of a confused person may not be completely beneficial if those hourly encounters cause agitation. Likewise, assisting a terminally ill man to die in his home may need to be reevaluated if it is causing his wife considerable physical and emotional strain. All variables must be considered in evaluating care.

Legal Considerations

Documentation. The medical record is a legal document that must be accurate and reflect actual occurrences. All entries should contain date, time, signature, and title of person making entry. Patient must give written consent for release of this documented information to sources other than agency staff. Other forms of written communication can carry liability such as articles, academic papers, correspondence (letters of reference, discharge summaries, publications).

Nursing Implications

- Remember that anything entered into that record can be used in a court of law; thus, entries should be correct, timely and conscientious.
- Do not use patient or agency names in writings for publication/distribution without obtaining written consent.
- Do not include information in correspondence statements that could be seen as defamatory or injurious to the reputation of an individual or agency.
- Do not alter documentation by changing dates, occurrences, or destroying and replacing original documentation.
- If fictitious or erroneous documentation is discovered or suspected, it should be brought to the immediate supervisor's attention promptly (preferably in writing).

Negligence. This consists of failure to take reasonable and prudent action so injury results.

Nursing Implications

- Avoid negligence by
  - doing only what equipped, skilled, and licensed to do
  - maintaining competency by keeping current of nursing practice
  - using good judgment; following acceptable standards of practice

- delegating carefully based on known capabilities of delegatee; following up on delegated tasks
- adhering closely to agency policies and procedures
- anticipating potential mishaps; working to reduce the risk of incidents occurring
- following medical orders as written
- questioning or refusing orders that appear incorrect
- actively observing and listening for patient's complaints, changes in patient's physical or mental status, equipment malfunction
- responding promptly to complaints or unusual occurrences
- documenting accurately and thoroughly

Invasion of Privacy.   This is the infringement of an individual's right to keep self and possessions from the public eye. Examples are

- releasing of information or record without patient's written permission
- allowing the presence of visitors, students, reporters, or others not directly involved with the patient's case during treatment
- presenting patient at a conference or meeting without permission
- displaying patient's deformity/incision/symptoms to unauthorized persons
- inadequately draping/protecting sedated, confused, or helpless patient
- using, without permission, patient's name, photograph, or other identifying information in an article, presentation, or advertisement

Nursing Implications

- Avoid invasion of privacy by respecting confidentiality of patient's record, nurse-client relationship.
- Do not release information concerning the patient to unauthorized persons (includes answering questions).
- Protect patient from unauthorized visitors (in room or treatment area).
- Obtain written permission before using patient's photograph or name in literature, conference presentations, etc.
- Take appropriate precautions to safeguard computer-stored information from unauthorized access.
- Follow agency's consent procedure, facilitate consent process by answering patient's questions honestly.

Consent.   Written consent demonstrates that the patient authorizes the care giver to perform specific procedures. Most facilities have a standard consent form which patients sign upon admission, authorizing routine and customary services. This consent does not cover all procedures, however. Special written consent should be obtained for

- surgery
- use of anesthesia
- moderate to high-risk diagnostic procedures
- use of cobalt or radiation

- electroshock therapy
- experimental drugs or procedures
- anything other than ordinary, routine care

Nursing Implications

Consent should be informed, in that patient fully understands the procedure. To assure that consent is informed

- outline on the consent form the name of the procedure, what it is used for, the steps that will occur, consequences, possible side effects, risks and alternatives.
- have a responsible professional obtain consent. The physician may delegate responsibility for obtaining consent but s/he remains liable.
- if the patient has been determined legally incompetent, obtain written consent from the legal guardian. If there is no legal judgment that the patient is incompetent, the patient has the right to grant or deny consent, regardless of staff's feelings about the patient's competency. When there is doubt that a legally competent patient understands the procedure, it may be a safeguard to obtain informed consent of the nearest relative in addition to the patient.

Telephone Orders.   Even when approved by agency policy, telephone orders involve many risks and can subject the nurse to liability for malpractice. If a recording device is used to record telephone orders the physician must be informed that the call is being recorded or the recording will not be admissible in court should there be legal action.

Nursing Implications

- Check agency policy regarding telephone orders and adhere to it strictly.
- Minimize the risks of accepting a telephone order by
    - ensuring telephone order is received directly from the physician by authorized staff, who are then responsible for it; do not accept second-hand messages from secretaries or assistants.
    - assuring adequate information has been communicated to the physician (e.g., patient's current status, vital signs, symptoms, medications, treatments, allergies); document it.
    - writing orders as given; read complete instructions back to the physician.
    - questioning or refusing to implement an order if it does not sound appropriate.
    - writing orders directly on the physician's order sheet, include date, time, physician's name, nurse's signature and title.
    - having every order signed by the physician according to policy or regulation.

Wills.   Wills are legal documents spelling out the desired disposition of a patient's property after death. They should be written with an attorney's assistance if at all possible. The most recently compiled will prevails at time of death. Conditions for legality include

- signed, dated, witnessed (required number of witnesses varies from state to state; witnesses cannot be beneficiaries)
- person must be mentally sound, able to independently determine preferred disposition of property, understand the implications of the will and what it says
- no evidence of fraud or coercion in will development

Nursing Implications

- Encourage all patients to draw up a will if they have not done so as this will avoid family conflict, expense after death and allow the individual, not the state, to decide how assets will be divided
- Alternatives to traditional wills such as holographic (handwritten) or oral wills may prove invalid if legal requirements for them within a given state are not fulfilled.
- Seek legal advice if patient's competence is in question.
- Do not witness a patient's will
  - might invalidate the document (legally)
  - nurse could be suspected of influencing the patient (due to patient dependency on the nurse for daily needs)
  - may violate agency policy (assure agency has policy regarding wills and follow it)
  - if no friend or family member (nonbeneficiary) is available to witness, seek an administration representative's assistance or an objective person such as an ombudsman.

Malpractice Insurance.   Questions to ask about your or your agency's policy include

- Does your employer carry a policy for you?
- Have you actually seen a copy of the policy?
- Is the policy effective only when you are working?
- What conditions must be met for coverage?
- What is covered? What is not?
- What are the limits for each claim?
- Will legal defense be covered?
- Can additional coverage be purchased?

Geriatric Services

Geriatric care services have been established to maintain optimal function of elderly individuals and to effectively manage problems within the geriatric population. Older patients should be able to move freely among services to meet their changing needs. Needs for service and assistance can range from very few needs to needs for complete care. A variety of services are available within the community and at facilities offering wide ranging services.

General

Information and Referral.   Local libraries, offices on aging, and health departments can direct the patient to an appropriate source of help, and serve as excellent resources for locating services in a specific community. State health care associations make referrals and are listed in the white pages of telephone books.

Financial Aid.   Local offices of the Social Security Administration and Department of Social Services determine eligibility for financial assistance and special benefits.

Banking.   Transportation and crime problems can be reduced by having Social Security and other checks managed by direct deposit. Many banks offer the elderly free checking and will assist in balancing checkbooks and managing bills.

Recreation.   Diversion and activity promote the health and well-being of the elderly. Local bureaus of recreation, religious groups, and service agencies sponsor senior centers and activities. Often, theaters, restaurants, and travel agencies provide special discounts for older adults.

Transportation.   Public transit agencies and local chapters of the Red Cross can provide or direct the patient to low-cost or handicapped transportation. Hospital social work departments may be able to assist with transportation for clinic visits.

Life Care.   For an initial fee and monthly payment, persons can enter a life-care community that will provide housing and services specific to the interests and needs of older adults. Health care also is included, usually ranging from wellness management through skilled nursing home care. Persons usually enter a life-care community when healthy, with intentions to spend their remaining years there. This arrangement usually provides for housing and various levels of health care as the patient's status changes.

When Minimal Assistance is Needed

Homemaker.   Public social service and private agencies can provide assistance with light housekeeping and shopping chores to help the elderly maintain independent living in the community.

Personal Care.   Bathing, dressing, and meal assistance may be required to aid the elderly in living at home. This form of care, which is less intense than home health (see below), can be obtained from public and private service agencies.

Home-delivered Meals.   Health departments, social service agencies, and religious organizations can provide or direct the patient to such services as "Meals on Wheels" in a specific community; these will usually provide one warm nutritious meal and a cold snack, delivered right to the patient's door.

Foster Care.   Social service departments can find placement for older persons who need room, board, and supervision in private homes.

Telephone Reassurance.   Homebound or at-risk elderly can obtain a daily social contact and safety check by having someone call them at a prearranged time.

When Moderate Assistance is Needed

Home Health Care.   A variety of public and private home health agencies may provide this level of service for patients who need skilled nursing services or special therapy, such as physical therapy or dialysis.

Day Care/Treatment Centers.   Patients are transported to these sites and receive health, social and recreational services for a portion of the day. The thrust of the program may be medical, social or psychiatric.

When Total Assistance is Needed

Institutional Care.   Nursing homes, chronic hospitals, and other long-term care facilities offer continuous services to patients when 24-hour care and supervision is needed. These institutions can serve as permanent or as a temporary care site until the patient's condition improves.

Combinations.   Frequently, very ill individuals can be cared for by the creative combination of multiple resources, e.g., a day-care program on weekdays, homemaker services on weekend days, and a private aide sleeping in during the night. Individual resources and the availability of community resources can determine what the possibilities for these arrangements can be.

The nurse needs to be aware of available resources and plan services carefully, coordinating measures to meet physical, emotional, and socioeconomic needs. Individualized plans are necessary to meet patient needs and preferences. Providing preventive, supportive services helps promote independence and can prevent development of problems.

Finances

Social Security was developed in 1935 as supplemental income for retired workers in old age. In 1939 the plan changed to include payments to certain dependents when the worker retired and to survivors if the worker died. More participants were allowed in the 1950s such as the self-employed, local and state employees, armed forces, clergy, household and farm employees. Disability insurance was added in 1954. Cost-of-living provision was enacted in 1972.

- Benefits (based on credits earned during work years)
  - one quarter of coverage is earned for each quarter of worker contribution
  - special provisions exist for surviving mothers and dependent children of deceased workers who have not earned sufficient credit
  - dependents of retired, disabled, or deceased workers, unmarried children under age 18 (or 22 if full time students); disabled children, dependent spouse over age 62 (or spouse under 62 caring for dependent children), divorced spouse (under certain conditions)

- Benefit calculation
    - family benefits based upon individual contributions; if both husband and wife qualify, benefits are calculated on the larger of the two amounts
    - a minimum benefit exists
    - benefits are reduced for retired workers under age 72 who return to work and earn above a specified amount

Medicare, a 1965 amendment to the Social Security Act (Title XVIII), provides medical insurance for persons age 65 or older. It is a federally-funded, standard coverage for all older persons regardless of their state of residence. Payment into the Social Security system assures institutional coverage at no cost; physician/outpatient coverage requires payment of a monthly premium. Medicare covers both institutional and physician/outpatient services such as

- hospital care
- skilled nursing home care committee
- hospice care
- physician services
- outpatient hospital services
- outpatient therapies
- outpatient surgery
- outpatient rehabilitation

NOTE: Since specific preconditions and limitations may exist for each service, patients should be advised to consult with an agency's Medicare resource/specialist or the local office of the Social Security Administration.

Medical Assistance (Medicaid), a 1965 amendment to the Social Security Act (Title XIX), provides medical insurance to low income persons of any age and is funded by state and federal contributions. For patients eligible for both services, Medical Assistance supplements Medicare coverage. The services vary from state to state but basic coverage includes

- inpatient hospital care
- outpatient hospital services
- laboratory and x-ray services
- physicians' services
- nursing home care
- home health care.

Nursing Implications

- Refer patients to the local department of social services to determine eligibility/benefits.
- To determine eligibility for various benefits, have patients contact the nearest social security office when they
    - are at least age 62 and within several months of retirement
    - are age 65 (retiring or not)
    - become disabled
    - experience the death of a family member who has received benefits

References

American Nurses Association. (1981). *A statement of the scope of gerontological nursing practice.* Kansas City, MO: American Nurses Association.

Anderson, F., & Williams, B. (1983). *Practical management of the elderly* (4th ed.). Boston: Blackwell Scientific Publications.

Baines, E. (1984). Medicare and Medicaid—differences and similarities. *Journal of Gerontological Nursing, 19*(1), 36-37.

Brock, A. (1984). Gerontological nursing in the 80's-flight or fight. *Journal of Gerontological Nursing, 10*(3), 102.

Burnside, I. (1983). Nursing and the aged. In F. Steinberg (Ed.), *Care of the geriatric patient* (6th ed.). St. Louis: Mosby.

Burnside, I. (1980). *Nursing and the aged* (2nd ed.). New York: McGraw-Hill.

Burnside, I. (1980). *Psychosocial nursing care of the aged* (2nd ed.). New York: McGraw-Hill.

Carnevali, D., & Patrick, M. (Eds.). (1979). *Nursing management for the elderly.* Philadelphia: Lippincott.

Carpenito, L. (1983). *Nursing diagnosis: Application to clinical practice.* Philadelphia: Lippincott.

Carpenito, L. (1984). *Handbook of nursing diagnosis.* Philadelphia: Lippincott.

Chung, S. (1983). Foot care. *Journal of Gerontological Nursing, 9,* 213.

Creighton, H. (1981). *Law every nurse should know* (4th ed.). Philadelphia: Saunders.

Davis, B. (1983). The gerontological nursing specialty. *Journal of Gerontological Nursing, 9*(10), 526-532.

Ebersole, P., & Hess, P. (1983). *Toward healthy aging: Human needs and nursing response* (2nd ed.). St. Louis: Mosby.

Eliopoulos, C. (1983). *Nursing administration of long term care.* Rockville, MD: Aspen Systems Corp.

Eliopoulos, C. (1979). *Gerontological nursing.* New York: Harper & Row.

Eliopoulos, C. (1984). *Health assessment of the older adult.* Menlo Park, CA: Addison-Wesley.

Eliopoulos, C. (1984). A self-care model for gerontological nursing. *Geriatric Nursing, 5,* 23-26.

Forbes, E., & Fitzsimons, V. (1981). *The older adult. A process for wellness.* St. Louis: Mosby.

Furukawa, C., & Shomkes, D. (1982). *Community health services for the aged.* Rockville, MD: Aspen Systems Corp.

Hirsch, C., Morris, R., & Moritz, A. (1979). *Handbook of legal medicine* (5th ed.). St. Louis: Mosby.

Kane, R. (1984). Long-term care: Policy and reimbursement. In C. Cassel & J. Walsh (Eds.), *Geriatric medicine, Vol II.* New York: Springer.

Koin, D. (1984). Access to health care. In C. Cassel & J. Walsh (Eds.), *Geriatric medicine, Vol II.* New York: Springer.

Lodge, M. (1984). *Professional practice for nurse administrators in long term care.* Kansas City, MO: American Nurses Association.

Mezey, M., Rauckhorst, L., & Stokes, S. (1980). *Health assessment of the older individual.* New York: Springer.

Morlin, D. (1983). Protective services: Legal aspects. In W. Reichel (Ed.), *Clinical aspects of aging* (2nd ed.). Baltimore: Williams & Wilkins.

Murray, R., Huelskoetter, M., & O'Driscoll, D. (1980). *The nursing process in later maturity.* Englewood Cliffs, NJ: Prentice-Hall.

O'Brien, C. (1982). *Adult day care: A practical guide.* Monterey, CA: Wadsworth.

Orem, D. (1980). *Nursing: Concepts of practice* (2nd ed.). New York: McGraw-Hill.

Reinhardt, A., & Quinn, M. (Eds.) (1979). *Current practice in gerontological nursing.* St. Louis: Mosby.

Rossman, I. (1978). Options for care of the aged sick. In W. Reichel (Ed.), *The geriatric patient.* New York: HP Publishing.

Rossman, I. (1983). Newer options for elderly patients other than institutionalization. In W. Reichel (Ed.), *Clinical aspects of aging* (2nd ed.). Baltimore: Williams & Wilkins.

Schwab, M. (1983). Professional nursing and the care of the aged. In W. Reichel (Ed.), *Clinical aspects of aging* (2nd ed.). Baltimore: Williams & Wilkins.

Stanley, B., et al. (1984). The elderly patient and informed consent. Empirical findings. *Journal of the American Medical Association. 252*(10), 1302-1306.

Steffl, B. (1984). Why gerontological nursing? In B. Steffl (Ed.), *Handbook of gerontological nursing.* New York: Van Nostrand Reinhold.

Wells, T. (1982). What does commitment to gerontological nursing really mean? *Journal of Gerontological Nursing, 8,* 434.

Wells, T. (1983). Hummm, huh, and ahha!: Gerontological nursing research. *Journal of Gerontological Nursing, 9,* 378.

Yurick, A., Robb, S., Spier, B., & Ebert, N. (1980). *The aged person and the nursing process.* New York: Appleton-Century-Crofts.

CHAPTER 2

AN OVERVIEW OF AGING

Facts About the Aging Population

Ours is an aging society both in the growing number of elderly people who comprise it and the older median age for the entire population. At the end of the 18th century the median age was 16 years; it now exceeds 30 years and by the year 2000 will be 35 years. Just 4% of the population was 65 years of age or older at the beginning of this century; now the portion of elderly exceeds 12% and will reach 20% by the year 2030. American life expectancy is increasing although differences between the sexes and races exist (Table 2.1). An obvious outcome of the life expectancy differences among the elderly is that women outnumber men in later years.

Age	Male to female ratio
Birth	10.5:10
65	7:10
85	5:10

The differences in life expectancy and the tendency for men to marry women younger than themselves (more than one-third of men over age 65

Table 2.1 U.S. Life Expectancies (1983)

White female	78.8 years
Non-white female	75.3 years
White male	71.6 years
Non-white male	67.1 years

Note: From "Vital Statistics of the U.S." by U.S. National Center for Health Statistics, 1985. *Statistical Abstract of the U.S.* (105th ed., No. 102), p 69. Washington, D.C.: U.S. Bureau of the Census.

have wives under age 65) accounts for the fact that most older men are married whereas most older women are widowed. There are five widows for every widower in old age.

Not only are more people reaching old age than ever before, but they are living longer after they reach their 65th birthday than did earlier generations (Table 2.2). Thus, the elderly population is becoming an older age group.

Health and the Aged.   Nearly 90% of all older persons suffer from a chronic illness. Chronic conditions are more than four times more prevalent in the elderly as in other age groups. More often than not, the older individual has several chronic illnesses for which medications and treatments must be juggled. Although acute conditions occur less frequently in later life, they are not to be considered minor problems. The elderly experience higher rates of complications and mortality from acute illnesses.

The leading causes of death for the age 65-and-over group are heart disease, cancer, and stroke. Almost one-half of the elderly have illnesses that interfere to some degree with their ability to engage in normal activities of daily living.

When the 10 leading causes of death are compared between the sexes, some differences can be found (Table 2.3). As can be noted in this list, accidents are a major threat to older persons. Sensorineural deficits and the effects of illnesses predispose the elderly to accidental injury. Although automobile related accidents are the most common cause of accidental death in the 65-to-74-year-old group, falls rank first as the most common fatal injury for the entire older population.

Finances.   In general, the elderly do not engage in a significant amount of preventive health care and screening. This may be due in part to the lack of insurance coverage for these practices.

Health care providers are in a cost-containment era that needs to control costs of the insurance programs that the elderly depend upon. In 1985 one in five Americans received Medicare or Medicaid benefits; 42 cents of every federal dollar was spent on programs for the elderly (particularly Social Security and Medicare); and two-thirds of older Americans' health care bills were paid by the government. As increasing numbers of people reach old

Table 2.2   Ages of the Older Population

Year	% of Older Population		
	65-74	75-84	85+
1900	71	25	4
1950	68	27	5
1975	62	30	8
2000	55	34	11

Note: From "Current Population Reports" 1983. Series P-25, Nos. 519, 704, and 721. Washington, D.C.: U.S. Bureau of the Census.

age and depend on these resources, concern develops regarding the system's ability to bear this burden (Table 2.4).

Despite what is claimed to be significant government assistance, the financial status of most older people is far from comfortable (Table 2.5). Social Security benefits, intended as a supplement to other sources of income, are the primary means of support for many. Only a minority of older adults receive private pension benefits; in fact, only approximately one-half of all current workers are enrolled in pension plans to assist them in their old age. Few elderly are employed, constituting only 4% of the total labor force. The

Table 2.3 Ten Leading Causes of Death for Population Age 65 Years and Over

Both Sexes	
Cause	*Number*
1. Heart disease	548,956
2. Malignant neoplasms	224,543
3. Cerebrovascular diseases	149,304
4. Influenza and pneumonia	48,405
5. Arteriosclerosis	28,032
6. Diabetes mellitus	24,797
7. Accidents	23,961
8. Bronchitis, emphysema, asthma	17,623
9. Cirrhosis of liver	8,378
10. Nephritis and nephrosis	5,732

Males		*Females*	
Cause	*Number*	*Cause*	*Number*
1. Heart disease	272,205	1. Heart disease	276,751
2. Malignant neoplasms	123,983	2. Malignant neoplasms	100,560
3. Cerebrovascular diseases	65,052	3. Cerebrovascular diseases	94,252
4. Influenza and pneumonia	24,307	4. Influenza and pneumonia	24,098
5. Bronchitis, emphysema, asthma		5. Arteriosclerosis	17,069
		6. Diabetes mellitus	15,524
6. Accidents	12,527	7. Accidents	11,434
7. Arteriosclerosis	10,963	8. Bronchitis, emphysema, asthma	
8. Diabetes mellitus	9,273		
9. Cirrhosis of liver	5,297	9. Cirrhosis of liver	3,801
10. Suicide	3,489	10. Nephritis and nephrosis	2,763

Note: From "Vital Statistics of the United States," 1981. Washington, D.C.: U.S. National Center for Health Statistics.

Table 2.4 Average Per Capita Health Care Expenditure

Age	*Per capita health care expenditure*
19-64	$ 764
65 and over	$2,026

Note: From "Age differences in health care spending," by C. Fisher, 1983. *Health Care Financing Review,* 1(4), pp 65-90.

fourth ranking means of support for the elderly is public assistance (Upp, 1982). Many elderly recipients of public assistance depend upon this means of support for the first time in their old age. They often become poor when they become old.

Home and Family.   Few individuals relocate to retirement communities or other locations in old age, remaining instead in the areas in which they have lived most of their lives. Compared to other age groups, there is a higher proportion of old people in rural areas. Few live in suburban areas, although the number may increase as the young adults who moved to suburbia in the 1950s and 1960s grow older.

Most elderly have strong ties with their families. Less than one-third have no families or live alone. Important assistance and support are exchanged between the elderly and their children. Although they have strong bonds, most elderly prefer to live separate from their offspring. Relationships between older spouses and siblings tend to strengthen and stabilize in late life.

Theories of Aging

For centuries there has been interest in explaining why and how human beings age. Although this mystery has yet to be solved, there are several theories that attempt to explain the aging process. They can be catagorized as *biologic* theories that address the anatomic and physiologic changes occurring with age, and *psychosocial* theories that explain the thought processes and behaviors of aging persons (Table 2.6)

Theories of aging are just that because the aging process is unique to each individual. There is no single factor known to be responsible for the aging process. Certain factors can interfere with healthy aging, such as poor nutrition, excessive exposure to ultraviolet light, pollution, inadequate stress management, and disease-producing organisms. Factors that can promote positive aging are a well-balanced diet, mental and physical activity, early detection and correction of health problems, and good hygiene.

Nursing Implications.   If the theories of aging do nothing else, they should help nurses understand the variety of factors that impact the aging process. This results in a unique style of aging in each individual. Just as differences exist between five-year-olds or 15-year-olds or 25-year-olds, no two 65-, 75-, or 85-year-olds will be identical either. In fact, with the many

Table 2.5   Average Household Income

Age	Average household income
19-64	$21,063
65 and over	$12,628

Note: From "Money income of households, families and persons in the U.S." 1982. *Current Population Reports*, Series P-60, No. 132. Washington, D.C.: U.S. Dept. of Commerce, Bureau of the Census.

Table 2.6 Theories of Aging

Factor	Hypothesis
Free radical structure	Parts of molecules break off or loose electron from these free parts attach to other molecules causing altered cellular structure. Environmental pollutants are believed to promote free radical activity. Some foods especially thought to reduce free radical activity are those rich in Vitamins A, C, and E.
Cross-link of collagen	Collagen constitutes 25%-30% of body protein and forms gelatin-like cell matrix. With age, collagen cross-links, becoming more insoluble and rigid. Some chemicals are thought to reduce cross-linkage (e.g., lathyrogens, prednisolene and penicillamine).
Programmed cells	Just as the body possesses an inherited biologic clock that triggers events such as the onset of puberty, cells are believed programmed to "age" at specific times.
Autoimmune reactions	Immunologic system loses capacity for self-regulation and begins perceiving normal or age-altered cells as foreign matter. The system reacts by forming antibodies to destroy those cells. A decline in the immunologic system is thought to allow the development of infections and cancer, and to play a role in the development of diseases such as diabetes mellitus, atherosclerosis, hypertension, and rheumatic heart disease.
Lipofuscin	Lipofuscin is a lipoprotein by-product of metabolism, not known to have any function in the body. With age, lipofuscin accumulates, particularly in the liver, heart, ovaries, and neurons. A relationship exists between age and the amount of accumulated lypofuscin. Other species have been found to accumulate lipofuscin.
Somatic mutation	Such factors as DNA alteration or RNA mutation(s), protein or enzyme synthesis cause defective cellular structure and function. With age defective cells multiply and lead to organ abnormalities, system dysfunction.
Stress	Repeated wear and tear impairs the efficiency of cellular function and eventually leads to physical decline.
Radiation	Laboratory studies reveal shorter lifespans in rats, mice, and dogs exposed to nonlethal radiation doses; it is thought that the same can occur in humans. This theory is supported by the fact that ultraviolet light is known to cause solar elastosis (wrinkling of skin caused by replacement of collagen by elastin) and promote skin cancer.
Nutrition	The quality and quantity of diet is thought to influence lifespan. Problems caused by obesity, cholesterol, and vitamin deficiencies support this theory.

Table 2.6 Theories of Aging (continued)

Factor	Hypothesis
Disengagement	Developed in late 1950s by Elaine Cummings and William Henry. Aging individuals and society gradually withdraw from each other for mutual benefit: societal activities can be transferred from old to young in orderly fashion and older persons are allowed time to focus on self with reduced social burdens. Theory's popularity undermined by the recognition that a) each individual has a different aging pattern and b) the process often damages both society and the aged.
Activity	Developed by Robert Havighurst in 1960s. Aging individuals should be expected to maintain norms of middle-aged adults: employment, activity, replacement of lost relationships. Age-related physical, mental, and socioeconomic losses may present legitimate obstacles to maintaining activity, thereby reducing universality of theory.
Development	Described by Bernice Neugarten in 1960s; longitudinal studies still being conducted. Basic personality, attitude, and behaviors remain constant throughout the lifespan. Allows multiple options for aging and recognizes the individuality of the aging process.

years of living they have experienced, elderly persons will probably show greater diversity than persons in other age groups. Astute assessment is needed to recognize the unique characteristics of the aged patient, and truly individualized care planning and delivery are crucial.

It is important to understand that nothing will eliminate or reverse the aging process. Immortality and eternal youth are not achievable. Patients should be advised to avoid fads that claim to stop aging or remove the effects of growing old.

Knowing that certain factors interfere with healthy aging it is important to avoid or minimize their impact. For example, some beneficial measures could include

- eating a nutritious diet low in carbohydrates and fats
- limiting exposure to ultraviolet light
- avoiding exposure to pollutants (e.g., noise, tobacco, drugs, polluted air and water)
- preventing infections and diseases; identifying and treating them early if they do occur
- managing stress effectively
- maintaining a physically and mentally active state

Physical Changes With Age

With age there is a gradual loss in the number of cells, so that by the time an individual reaches age 70 there are 30% fewer cells in the body. Because older bodies are not reduced in size by 30% a compensatory measure must exist. The cells enlarge in size so that fewer but larger cells comprise the body, making its total mass appear relatively unaltered. The many alterations in organ function result from these basic changes on the cellular level.

The cells are of irregular structure. The fluid within the cell decreases although extracellular fluid and plasma volume remain constant. The reduction in intracellular fluid results in less total body fluid, which causes dehydration to be a greater risk.

There is a loss of tissues throughout the body with the exception of adipose tissue. A higher proportion of the body's composition is fat, a consideration in nutritional assessment and drug therapy since certain drugs are stored in adipose tissue. The loss of subcutaneous tissue is evidenced through a deepening of the hollows of intercostal and supraclavicular spaces, orbits and axillae, and sagging breasts. Reduced subcutaneous tissue causes less natural insulation and a more severe response to temperature fluctuation.

Some of the other general changes in body composition include progressive decrease in serum albumin, increase in globulin, a slow increase in serum cholesterol throughout adulthood and a stabilization or slight decrease after the sixth decade, decreased ability to metabolize glucose, and higher blood glucose levels in the absence of diabetes.

Cardiovascular.   Normally, the size of the heart does not change with age; the enlarged hearts frequently noted in older persons are associated with cardiac disease, not normal aging. The valves become thick and rigid due to sclerosis and fibrosis. As a compensatory measure for less efficient oxygen utilization, the aortic volume and systolic blood pressure rise.

Decreased efficiency of the heart muscle reduces cardiac output by approximately 1% per year during adulthood. Although this does not significantly affect the resting heart rate, profound effects are noted under stressful conditions when it takes the heart longer to return to a normal rate. There is greater peripheral resistance in vessels caused by calcium deposits, cross linking of collagen, and a reduction in elastin. Capillary walls are thicker, which may impede the effective exchange of nutrients and promote capillary fragility.

Pulmonary.   The lungs lose elasticity and become more rigid resulting in approximately a 50% increase in residual capacity between youth and old age, a lower vital capacity, decreased maximum breathing capacity, and a greater likelihood of collapse during opening of chest cavity or pneumothorax.

Alveoli are fewer in number and larger in size. Alveolar ducts and bronchioles have an increased diameter. There is less ciliary activity. The anteroposterior chest diameter increases. As a result, the thoracic transverse measurement may be reduced and some kyphosis noted. Costal cartilage calcification and partial contraction of the inspiratory muscles cause decreased mobility of the ribs. Weaker thoracic inspiratory and expiratory muscles create conditions that promote respiratory infections, including incomplete lung expansion, insufficient basilar inflation, decreased ability to expel foreign or accumulated material, and inefficient cough response.

Blood oxygen level (pO_2) decreases by 10%-15%. Though blood carbon dioxide level (pCO_2) remains constant, the high prevalence in the elderly of chronic obstructive lung disease, which raises pCO_2 levels, frequently causes higher levels to be found. Oxygen utilization under stress is reduced due to delayed oxygen diffusion, ineffective perfusion, and inefficient utilization of oxygen by stressed tissues.

Gastrointestinal.   Teeth are not normally lost as a result of aging although past dental health and dietary practices have caused more than 50% of today's elderly to be edentulous. Periodontal disease becomes the number one cause of tooth loss after age 30. If natural teeth exist they tend to have flatter surfaces, stains, and varying degrees of erosion and abrasion of the crown and root structure. Teeth that are loose or break easily can be aspirated, creating the risk of lung infections and abscesses.

Approximately one-third the volume of saliva as produced in youth is produced in old age, thus the mixing and swallowing of food, tablets, and capsules can be difficult without ample fluid intake. The decreased secretion of salivary ptyalin interferes with the digestion of starch. Atrophy of the epithelial covering occurs in the oral mucosa.

In late life approximately one-third the number of taste buds per papilla remain, which causes the taste threshold to increase. Pipe smoking causes a more profound loss. The receptors for sweet and salty flavors are effected most, thus food distastes can result.

Aspiration of food becomes of greater risk because of a weaker gag reflex, delayed emptying of the esophagus due to its slight dilation and decreased peristalsis, relaxation of the lower esophageal sphincter, and reduced stomach motility and emptying. This supports the need for smaller volumes of food to be consumed at each meal and the patient to remain in an upright position during and approximately 30 minutes after meals.

Hunger contractions are reduced due to less motor activity in the stomach. In addition, within the stomach there is thinner mucosal lining, less production of digestive juices (hydrochloric acid, pepsin, pancreatic enzymes), and reduced tolerance for fats, believed to be associated with decreased lipase production.

Some atrophy occurs along the small and large intestines. The internal anal sphincter is believed to lose its tone although research in this area is inconclusive at present. The elderly are predisposed to constipation as a result of decreased colonic peristalis and slower and duller neural impulses, which dull the signal to defecate.

The liver decreases in weight and storage capacity. There is a higher incidence of gallstones due to less efficient cholesterol stabilization and absorption. Although the levels remain adequate for digestive functions, there is a reduction in the volume and concentration of pancreatic enzymes. The pancreas gains more fat content.

Genitourinary.   Decreased tissue growth, a loss of nephrons, and athero-sclerosis causes the renal mass to become smaller with age. The function of the kidneys is altered by reduction in glomerular filtration rate (nearly 50% between youth and old age), a 50% decrease in renal blood flow resulting from a lower filtration rate, and a decline in tubular function causing less effective concentration of urine and a decreased reabsorption of glucose from the filtrate. These changes create problems in the filtration of drugs from the blood stream, as well as in the use of the urine specimen as a reliable screening tool.

Decreased bladder capacity and a delayed micturition reflex create problems for the elderly in urinary frequency, urgency, and nocturia. Urinary retention is more prevalent among the elderly. Incontinence is not a normal outcome of aging although many women (particularly those who have carried several pregnancies) experience stress incontinence due to a weakening of the pelvic diaphragm.

A majority of older men have some degree of prostatic enlargement, which increases urinary frequency. Most of this hypertrophy is benign but it produces a greater risk of malignancy, thus regular evaluation is essential.

Male reproductive changes include

- decreased testosterone production
- reduced sperm count
- smaller testes
- lower viscosity of seminal fluid
- need for more direct physical stimulation to achieve an erection; lessened ability to regain erection after interruption or completed intercourse

Female reproductive system changes include

- decreased estrogen production
- reduction in breast tissue
- shrinkage of uterus
- more alkaline vaginal secretions, increasing the risk of vaginitis
- narrowing, shortening, and increased fragility of vaginal canal
- drier vaginal canal necessitating longer foreplay or use of lubricant to facilitate penile penetration (if a lubricant is used it should be water based to prevent obstruction of the urethra)

There is no change in libido in either sex.

Musculoskeletal.   The muscles experience a loss of cells, overall mass, strength, and movement. Muscle tremors often occur, believed to be associated with degeneration of the extrapyramidal system. Bones become brittle and easy to fracture as a result of a gradual resorption of interior surface of long bones and slower new bone production on outside surface. There is a deterioration of the cartilage surface of joints, which limits joint activity and range of motion. Between ages 20 and 70 there is approximately a 2-inch reduction in height due to thinner intervertebral disks, shortening of vertebral column associated with cartilage loss, and slight kyphosis and flexion of the hips and knees.

Neurologic.   Nerve cells are lost with age and there is a lower nerve conduction velocity. The response to multiple stimuli and kinesthetic sense is reduced. Most reflexes are slowed, although deep tendon reflexes are retained. Stages 3 and 4 of sleep become less prominent. It is not unusual for sleep to be frequently interrupted; however, the actual amount of sleep loss is minimal.

Sensory.   The effects of aging on vision are profound, including

- presbyopia, a farsightedness that begins in the fourth decade and causes most people to require corrective lenses
- narrowing of visual field
- smaller pupil size, reducing visual adaptation to darkness
- yellowing of the lens, distorting low tone colors such as blues, greens, and violets
- opacity of the lens, causing glare to be a greater problem
- less efficient resorption of intraocular fluid, increasing the risk of glaucoma
- distorted depth perception
- development of arcus senilis (a partial or complete glossy white circle around the periphery of the iris)
- reduced lacrimal secretions, allowing eyes to become irritated more easily
- diminished olfaction, creating a safety hazard and reducing pleasurable awareness of the environment

Hearing also undergoes serious changes that can threaten the elderly's maintenance of a safe and normal life-style. Presbycusis is the term used to describe the age-related hearing loss that involves a dysfunction in the ability to transmit nerve impulses from the ear to the brain. Initially, high-frequency sounds (e.g., s, sh, ph, and ch) are filtered from the speech; as the condition progresses, middle and low frequencies are impacted. Hearing can be mechanically blocked by cerumen, which contains more keratin (making it harder) and accumulates.

There is an increased threshold for pain and touch. Conditions causing severe pain in younger persons can cause only minor pain or a sense of pressure in the elderly. The reduced ability to feel pressure increases the risk of skin breakdown. Alterations in proprioception (sense of physical position) can cause problems with balance and spatial orientation.

Integumentary.   With age the skin becomes less elastic, drier, and more fragile as wrinkling and sagging demonstrate. The risk of skin breakdown increases. "Age spots" or "liver spots" develop as a result of clustering of melanocytes. Excessive pigmentation can occur in areas exposed to the sun. Scalp, pubic, and axilla hair thins and loses color while hair in the nose and ears thickens. Women may find that they develop facial hair. Fingernails grow at a slower rate and become thick and brittle.

Endocrine.   The pituitary gland loses weight and vascularity, and contains increased amounts of connective tissue. Although there is an increase in follicle-stimulating hormone (FSH) in women there are no changes in male FSH, adrenocorticotropic hormone (ACTH), antidiuretic hormone (ADH), thyroid stimulating hormone (FSH), luteinizing hormone (LH), and growth hormone (GH).

A variety of changes impact the thyroid gland. Fibrosis, cellular infiltration, and increased modularity occur. A decrease in plasma T3 (plasma T4 is unchanged) is seen as well as a reduction in radioiodine accumulation, and a lower basal metabolic rate.

There is a delayed release of insulin by the beta cells of the pancreas. Some reduced peripheral sensitivity to circulating insulin is also thought to occur. Increased blood glucose levels in nondiabetic older persons are not uncommon and necessitate age-adjusted gradients for interpreting glucose tolerance tests.

The adrenal glands in old age are characterized by increased amounts of connective tissue; reduced lipid, pigmentation, cortical nodules; and reductions in secretion of cortisol (the plasma level of ACTH is normal). Blood level and urinary excretion of aldosterone, adrenal androgen production, and epinephrine and norepinephrine (although research supporting this is inconclusive at present) are also increased.

Ovarian-produced estrogen ceases after menopause; there is no significant change in adrenal-produced estrogen. Progesterone production and excretion are decreased. Testosterone production and metabolic clearance rates decline. Evidence is inconclusive regarding changes in blood testosterone levels. Less parathyroid stimulating hormone (PTH) is secreted by the parathyroid gland.

Implications of Changes.   The variety of physical changes experienced with normal aging can increase the risk of multiple health problems. Nurses must identify these risks and the possible nursing diagnoses that could be associated with them so that health problems can be prevented or, if present, effectively managed.

Psychologic Changes With Age

Personality.   There is no stereotypical profile of an older person. People do not become wise, feeble, childlike, rigid, or cantankerous in old age. Their basic psychologic characteristics will remain with them throughout their lives, resulting in diversity in psychologic status in advanced age. Personality changes in old age can be associated with physical or mental health problems.

Intelligence.   Basic intelligence is maintained. The wise old person most likely was always bright, while mentally dull elderly may have never had a high IQ. A decline in intelligence in old age usually is associated with a disease process and is not be be considered normal. Verbal comprehension and arithmetic abilities are unchanged. There is some decline in decoding ability, arrangement of geometric forms, spatial perception, and psychomotor performance.

IQ test performance may be hindered due to sensory deficits or the stress of being tested. These factors should be compensated for when assessing intelligence.

Memory.   Long-term memory does not change significantly. Short-term memory is poorer. A poor health status can weaken both short- and long-term memory.

Learning.   Past learning experiences and attitudes affect learning capacity in old age. There is a slower learning process, and health problems and stress can interfere with learning.

"Senility."   The word *senility* is a meaningless catch-all term that does a disservice to the elderly. People do not lose their minds or become mentally incapacitated as a result of normal aging. Mental dysfunction is an abnormality that deserves competent evaluation and intervention. At no time must impaired mental function be accepted as a normal condition of aging.

Developmental Tasks.   Each stage of life possesses challenges, needs, and problems, known as developmental tasks. If successfully completed these tasks can bring satisfaction and growth. When they are not met with success the result may be unhappiness and maladjustment. Most of the developmental tasks involve coping with daily life, adjusting to changes and losses, and coming to terms with one's own mortality. A variety of theories have been formulated to describe the developmental tasks of late life.

The work of Erik Erikson (1963) has become a classic in understanding the developmental tasks of each stage of life. Erikson claimed that the completion of developmental tasks could result in positive or negative outcomes that would affect one's entire life, i.e., unmet needs from one stage of life could interfere with successful completion of later stages. The stages and potential results are outlined in Table 2.7.

In the last stage of life, Erikson believed that the individual needs to meet the challenge of putting one's life in perspective, accepting the realities experienced and feeling as though one's life had meaning and usefulness. Despair would result from feelings of frustration or dissatisfaction with the life lived and the realization that it is too late to start over.

Robert Peck (1956) built upon and refined Erikson's work to offer three specific issues confronted in old age.

- Ego differentiation *vs.* role preoccupation, in which new roles are established to substitute for lost ones.
- Body transcendence, in which pleasures and mental activities minimize physical declines and disabilities.

Table 2.7 Developmental Stages

Stage of Life	Developmental Tasks		
Infancy	Trust	vs.	Mistrust
Toddler	Autonomy	vs.	Shame
Early childhood	Initiative	vs.	Guilt
Middle childhood	Industry	vs.	Inferiority
Adolescence	Identity	vs.	Identity diffusion
Adulthood	Intimacy	vs.	Isolation
Middle age	Generativity	vs.	Self-absorption
Old age	Integrity	vs.	Despair

- Ego transcendence *vs.* ego preoccupation, in which one's past and the value of one's current life supersede thoughts of one's impending death.

The functions of adjusting to losses and changes and meeting new challenges in late life were described by J.H. Barrett (1977) as either regressive or compensatory tasks. Regressive tasks include accepting physical decline, reduced sexuality, altered dependence-independence patterns, and a shrinking social world. Compensatory tasks include developing new leisure activities and work skills, and adjusting to altered environment, status, societal mores, and self-concept. Robert Butler and Myrna Lewis (1982) describe tasks of the elderly to be learning to live with infirmities, gaining satisfaction from the life lived, and preparing for death.

The developmental tasks of late life were catagorized by Priscilla Ebersole (1976) into three groups.

- Receptive tasks: Power and capacity in physical, social, cultural, and intellectual realms are relinquished and a certain amount of dependency accepted.
- Expressive tasks: A self-transcending philosophy is developed as older persons gain an appreciation for their place in life and the legacy they will leave.
- Dynamic tasks: This entails not only one's own physical and psychologic dying process but helping others learn about death.

The common themes throughout each of these descriptions of developmental tasks are that the elderly must adjust to significant changes, find meaning to their existence, and prepare for death. The nurse must appreciate that these major challenges are faced at a time when physical, emotional, and social reserves are reduced. Support and guidance are necessary to help the elderly meet the developmental tasks of old age in a satisfying and meaningful way.

References

Atchley, R. (1983). *Aging: Continuity and change.* Belmont, CA: Wadsworth.
Atchley, R. (1980). *The social forces in later life* (3rd ed.). Belmont, CA: Wadsworth.

Barrett, J. (1972). *Gerontological psychology*. Springfield, IL: Thomas.

Behnke, J., Finch, C., & Moment, G. (Eds.). (1978). *The biology of aging*. New York: Plenum.

Brock, A. (1984). From wife to widowhood: A changing lifestyle. *Journal of Gerontological Nursing, 10*(4), 8-15.

Butler, R., & Lewis, M. (1982). *Aging and mental health* (3rd ed.). St. Louis: Mosby.

Champlin, L. (1983). Early retirement: A catalyst for health problems? *Geriatrics, 38*(7), 106-109.

Check, J. (1984). How elders view learning. *Geriatric Nursing, 5*(1), 37-39.

Ebersole, P. (1976). Developmental tasks in later life. In I. Burnside (Ed.), *Nursing and the aged*. New York: McGraw-Hill.

Eisdorder, C., & Wilke, F. (1977). Stress, disease, aging, and behavior. In J. Birren & K. Schaie (Eds.), *Handbook for the psychology of aging*. New York: Van Nostrand Reinhold.

Erikson, E. (1963). *Childhood and society* (2nd ed.). New York: W.W. Norton.

Few, A., & Getty, R. (1967). Occurrence of lipofuscin as related to aging in the canine and porcine nervous system. *Journal of Gerontology, 22*, 357-367.

George, L. (1980). *Role transitions in later life*. Monterey, CA: Brooks/Cole.

Getty, C., & Humphreys, W. (Eds.). (1981). *Understanding the family: Stress and change in American family life*. New York: Appleton-Century-Crofts.

Goldman, R. (1984). Normal human aging: A theroretical context. In C. Cassel & J. Walsh (Eds.), *Geriatric medicine*, Vol. I. New York: Springer.

Goulet, L., & Baltes, P. (Eds.). (1979). *The theory and status of life span research*. New York: Academic Press.

Hayflick, L. (1977). The cellular basis for biological aging. In C. Finch & L. Hayflick (Eds.), *Handbook of the biology of aging*. New York: Van Nostrand Reinhold.

Havighurst, R. (1972). *Developmental tasks and education*. New York: David McKay.

Hernon, J. (1984). Exploding aging myths through retirement counseling. *Journal of Gerontological Nursing, 10*(4), 31-33.

Herr, J., & Weakland, J. (1979). *Counseling elders and their families*. New York: Springer.

Hess, B. (1976). *Growing old in America*. New Brunswick, NJ: Transaction Books.

Manney, J. (1975). *Aging in American society*. Detroit: University of Michigan, Wayne State University Institute of Gerontology.

Manuel, R. (Ed.). (1982). *Minority aging: Sociological and social psychological issues*. Westport, CT: Greenwood Press.

McLaughlin, F. (1983). Volunteerism and life satisfaction in old people: A test of the activity theory (abstract). *Gerontology, 23*(69)(special issue).

Meier, D. (1984). The cell biology of aging. In C. Cassel, & J. Walsh, (Eds.), *Geriatric medicine, Vol I*. New York: Springer.

Peck, R. (1956). Psychological developments in the second half of late life. In J. Anderson (Ed.), *Psychological aspects of aging*. Washington, DC: American Psychological Association.

Rockstein, M., & Sussman, M. (1977). *Biology of aging*. New York: Van Nostrand Reinhold.

Sinex, F. (1977). The molecular genetics of aging. In C. Finch & L, Hayfleck (Eds.), *Handbook of the biology of aging*. New York: Van Nostrand Reinhold.

Shock, N. (1977). Systems integration. In C. Finch, & L. Hayflick (Eds.), *Handbook of the biology of aging*. New York: Van Nostrand Reinhold.

Special Report on Aging (1981). Public Health Service, NIH Pub. No. 31-2328. NIA, Washington, DC: U.S. Dept. of Health and Human Services,

Storandt, M. (1982). Psychological aspects. In F. Steinburg (Ed.), *Cowdry's the care of the geriatric patient* (6th ed.). St. Louis: Mosby.

Strieb, F. (1983). Two views of retirement: In the clinic and in the community. In W. Reichel (Ed.), *Care of the geriatric patient in the tradition of E.V. Cowdry* (6th ed.). St. Louis: Mosby.

Talbert, G. (1977). Aging of the reproductive system. In C. Finch & L. Hayflick (Eds.), *Handbook of the biology of aging*. New York: Van Nostrand Reinhold.

Thompson, M. (1984). *The care of the elderly in general practice*. New York: Churchill Livingstone.

U.S. Department of Health, Education and Welfare. (1978). *Changes—Research on aging and the aged.* (DHEW Publication No. NIH-78-85). Washington, DC: U.S. Government Printing Office.

Upp, M. (1982). A look at the economic status of the aged then and now. *Social Security Bulletin,* (March), 16-22.

CHAPTER 3

DRUGS: SPECIAL CONSIDERATIONS IN THE ELDERLY

Drug use in the elderly population is a significant concern. The high prevalence of chronic diseases in this age group contributes to high drug use. It is the rare older person who is not taking some medication; typically, several medications are taken concurrently. Studies have shown that nursing home residents have an average of six drugs prescribed, with some receiving as many as 23 different medications. Although they represent 12% of the population, the elderly receive approximately 25% of all prescription drugs. The elderly are frequently prescribed drugs when nonpharmacologic means of treatment could be utilized. It is less time consuming for the provider to offer a drug than to teach or try alternative approaches. Consumers contribute to the problem by expecting a prescription whenever they visit the physician with a complaint. Over-the-counter drugs are easily available for a variety of the problems elderly persons experience. Often, the hazards and special precautions associated with the use of these drugs is not known by the older consumer, and additional problems can be created.

The elderly react differently to drug therapy (see Table 3.1). Dosages acceptable for middle-aged persons can be excessive for older adults and accumulate to toxic levels. Adverse reactions occur more frequently and may present an atypical picture. A change in mental status can be the first clue of a drug reaction in the elderly (Table 3.2). However, this is often not recognized by the staff due to acceptance of confusion or disorientation so frequently presumed in the elderly.

Table 3.1 Age-Related Changes Affecting Drug Therapy in the Elderly

Change	Impact	Nursing Measure
Drier mucous membrane of oral cavity	Tablets and capsules may stick to roof or sides of mouth and not be swallowed; they can dissolve in and irritate mouth.	Offer fluids before drug administration to moisten mouth and ample fluids during administration. Inspect mouth or advise patient to inspect mouth for any tablet or capsule that may not have been swallowed (the presence of dentures and reduced sensations may cause the patient to be unaware of the presence of the medication). Unless contraindicated, break large tablets to facilitate swallowing.
Decreased circulation to lower bowel and vagina; lower body temperature	Suppositories may have difficulty melting, risk being expelled.	Explore possibility of using alternative route. Allow longer time for suppository to melt. Check, or advise patient to check, that suppository has melted before getting out of bed to resume activities.
Decreased tissue elasticity; reduced muscle mass and activity	Poor seal of tissues after injection, oozing; poor absorption	Use upper, outer quadrant of buttocks for IM injections and rotate sites. Use Z-track injection technique for all injections to facilitate sealing. Cleanse skin from any medication that has oozed to its surface.
Decreased pain sensation	Infection or other problem at injection site may not be detected.	Check injection sites regularly.
Decreased cardiac efficiency	Circulatory overlaod during IV administration of medications is of greater risk.	Monitor IV drip closely. Observe for signs of circulatory overload (rise in blood pressure, rapid respirations, coughing, shortness of breath).
Less gastric acid	Slower absorption of drugs	Ensure gastric acid is not further reduced by other drugs (e.g., antacids).
Increase in adipose tissue compared to total body mass	Certain drugs that are stored in adipose tissue (e.g., diazepam, chlorpromazine) will accumulate and remain in the body for a longer duration.	Ensure dosages are age-adjusted. Become familiar with the adverse efects of drugs administered and observe for these effects.

Table 3.1   Age-Related Changes Affecting Drug Therapy in the Elderly (continued)

Change	Impact	Nursing Measure
Reduction in number of functioning nephrons; decreased glomerular filtration rate; reduced blood flow to kidneys	Biologic half-life of drugs is extended; drugs take longer to be filtered from body; increased risk of adverse reactions.	Ensure age-adjusted dosages are prescribed.
Less production of liver enzymes	Slower metabolism of drugs; increased risk of adverse reactions	Observe for signs of adverse effects and obtain prompt treatment. (Be aware that altered mental status may be an initial manifestation of an adverse reaction.)

Nursing Management

Assessment

- Determine if nonpharmacologic approaches can solve or control the problem, e.g.,
  - warm milk and a backrub instead of a sedative
  - coffee or cranberry juice instead of a diuretic
  - warm soaks or position change instead of an analgesic
  - dietary change instead of an antacid or laxative
  - diversional activity instead of antipsychotic

- Ensure the lowest possible dosage is prescribed
  - the longer biologic half-life of most drugs in older persons warrants lower dosages
  - assess dosage in regard to body weight and known organ function

- Review other drugs being used for potential interactions.
- Keep a drug reference handy; with the growing number and changing knowledge of drugs it is unrealistic to expect to commit all drug facts to memory.
- Obtain specific guidelines for use of PRN medications and use them appropriately.
- Request that orders state the conditions for use (e.g., for pain, for fever above 100°, rather than an order for 2 tablets of aspirin).
- If patient must self-administer drugs, evaluate his/her capacity to do so (e.g., motor dexterity to manipulate container, knowledge, memory, judgment, vision, tendency to abuse drug).

Interventions

- Determine the best time of day to administer the medication (e.g., diuretics in the early morning, drugs that cause drowsiness at bedtime).

Table 3.2   Side Effects of Selected Drugs

	Abnormal bruising and bleeding	Acid-base imbalance	Acute excitement	Agitation	Anaphylactic Reaction	Anemias	Anorexia	Anxiety	Bone marrow depression	Breast enlargement with milk formation	Confusion	Convulsions	Delerium	Depression	Diarrhea	Disorientation	Dizziness	Drug fever	Dysrhythmias	Edema	Eye rolling	Fainting	Fluctuating blood glucose levels	GI disturbances	Hair loss	Hallucinations	"Hangover" effect	Headache	Hepatitis	Hives	Hypertension	Hypotension	Impaired renal function	Increased appetite	Indigestion	Inflamed pancreas	Intestinal obstruction
Acetaminophen	x				x	x																								x							
Amitriptyline			x								x	x	x				x	x	x			x	x			x					x	x		x			
Antacids		x																		x											x			x			x
Chloral Hydrate												x														x		x							x		
Chlordiazepoxide		x									x			x			x					x				x											
Chlorpromazine										x	x	x						x											x			x		x		x	
Diazepam		x									x						x					x															
Digoxin											x				x													x		x							
Fluphenazine			x							x							x											x	x								
Haloperidol			x		x	x	x			x	x			x	x	x				x		x		x		x		x									
Hydrochlorothiazide			x		x		x			x							x	x					x					x	x								x
Insulin											x												x														
Isoniazid										x	x		x				x	x										x									
Methyldopa				x																													x				
Perphenazine										x			x															x	x	x							
Phenobarbital									x			x	x		x		x	x								x		x	x	x							
Phenytoin						x					x		x				x	x										x	x					x			
Potassium Chloride															x									x													
Reserpine	x										x	x																									
Rifampin									x						x		x							x				x		x							
Theophylline								x			x				x		x		x									x									
Thioridazine			x			x		x	x	x	x													x				x									
Trifluoperazine			x								x							x																			
Trihexyphenidyl											x							x																			

• Identify special precautions for administration (e.g., relationship to meals or other drugs, whether an antagonist should be readily available).

• Give medication as prescribed, following any special instructions or precautions.

• Educate patient and patient's care givers about drugs and their purposes, administration, special precautions, and adverse reactions.

• Discuss with physician the possibility of drug holidays (Table 3.3) for the many benefits this plan provides; recognize that some physicians are unaware of this option and need to be informed of the possibilities.

• Observe if the drug is achieving the desired effect and whether side effects are occurring; document patient's response to drug therapy.

	Irritation of Tongue	Jaundice	Kidney stone formation	Lethargy	Lowered resistance to infection	Low grade fever	Muscle spasms	Nausea	Nightmares	Palpitations	Parkinson-like disorders	Peripheral Neuritis	Rash	Reduced platelets	Reduced WBC	Restlessness	Sexual impairment	Sleepwalking	Slurred speech	Stomach ulcers	Swelling: face and tongue	Swelling: glands	Swelling and tenderness of gums	Swelling: testicles	Swelling: vocal cords	Tachycardia	Temperature decrease	Temperature increase	Thought disturbances	Tingling sensations	Tremors	Unsteady gait	Vivid dreaming	Vision disturbances	Vomiting	Weakness
Acetaminophen													×		×																					
Amitriptyline	×						×		×	×	×		×			×					×			×							×	×			×	×
Antacids			×				×	×																											×	
Chloral Hydrate							×						×					×																	×	
Chlordiazepoxide	×			×			×						×						×															×	×	
Chlorpromazine						×	×			×			×													×										
Diazepam							×	×					×			×																			×	
Digoxin			×										×																						×	
Fluphenazine											×		×															×								
Haloperidol	×						×		×	×			×															×							×	×
Hydrochlorothiazide													×																						×	
Insulin																																				
Isoniazid													×									×									×	×			×	
Methyldopa			×										×																							×
Perphenazine							×			×			×															×								
Phenobarbital												×	×		×					×														×		
Phenytoin							×	×					×						×			×	×											×		
Potassium Chloride							×						×																						×	
Reserpine							×			×			×				×														×				×	
Rifampin													×	×														×					×		×	
Theophylline							×						×						×							×								×		
Thioridazine							×			×			×															×	×						×	
Trifluoperazine						×	×			×			×					×																	×	
Trihexyphenidyl							×						×																							

- Regularly question if the drug needs to be continued; if it is no longer needed or is ineffective, relay your observations to the physicians who rely on nurses to give them feedback concerning patient's responses to medication.
- Include family members in the evaluation process of effectiveness of medication since they are often the best judge of a change in behavior.

NOTE: Various drug groups are discussed throughout the book with the medical problems for which they are used. Table 3.4 references the location of these discussions.

Table 3.3   Drug Holidays

A drug holiday is the planned omission of a specific medication on one or more days each week.

Benefits
  Reduced risk of drug accumulating to toxic level in bloodstream
  Increased mental alertness
  Fewer restrictions on activities
  Cost savings
  Decreased demand on staff time

Requirements
  Interdisciplinary support and planning
  Thoughtful assessment of appropriate patients
  Careful selection of drugs
  Educate patient and family
  Stablized blood levels for certain drugs

Drugs not usually omitted
  Antibiotics
  Anticoagulants
  Anticonvulsants
  Hypoglycemic agents
  Insulin
  Ophthalmic drops

Table 3.4   Drug Groups Discussed In This Book

Drug Group	Discussed on Page(s)
Analgesics	215
Antacids	84
Antianginals	145
Antianxiety	230
Antidysrhythmics	136
Antibiotics	62
Anticoagulants	148
Antidepressants	227
Antidiabetics	80
Antihypertensives	147
Anti-inflammatories	165
Antipsychotics	194
Cardiac glycosides	137
Diuretics	135
Laxatives	101

References

Albrick, J. (1984). Geriatric pharmacology. In G. Schwartz, G. Bosker, & J. Grigsley (Eds.), *Geriatric emergencies.* Bowie, MD: Brady.

Avron, J. (1983). More on drugs and the elderly. *Long Term Care Administrator, 17*(5).

Berlinger, W. (1984). Adverse drug reactions in the elderly. *Geriatrics, 39*(5), 45-58.

Donlon, P., Schaffer, C., Eriksen, S., Pepitone-Rockwell, E., & Schaffer, L. (1983). *A manual of psychotropic drugs—A mental health resource.* Bowie, MD: Brady.

Greenblatt, D., Sellers, E., & Shoder, R. (1982). Drugs therapy: Drug disposition in old age. *New England Journal of Medicine, 306,* 1081-1088.

Jernigan, J. (1984). Update on drugs and the elderly. *American Family Physician, 5*(4), 238-247.

Keenan, R., Redsharo, A., Munson, J., & Mundt, W. (1983). The benefits of a drug holiday. *Geriatric Nursing, 4*(2), 103-104.

Lamy, P. (1982). *Prescribing for the elderly.* Boston: John Wright, PSG.

Lamy, P. (1983). Use of hypnotics in the elderly. *American Family Physician, 30*(2), 187-191.

Myers, M., Meier, D., & Walsh, J. (1984). General principles of pharmacology. In C. Cassel & J. Walsh (Eds.), *Geriatric medicine, Vol I.* New York: Springer.

Oppeneer, J., & Vervoren, T. (1983). *Gerontological pharmacology. A resource for health practitioners.* St. Louis: Mosby.

Portnoi, V., & Johnson, J. (1982). Tardive dyskinesia. *Geriatric Nursing, 3*(6), 39-40.

Roffham, D. (1984). Special concerns of digitalis use in older patients. *Geriatrics, 39*(6), 97-105.

Simonson, W. (1984). *Medications and the elderly. A guide for promoting proper use.* Rockville, MD: Aspen Systems.

Smith, W., & Steele, T. (1983). Avoiding diuretic-related complications in older patients. *Geriatrics, 38*(X), 117-119, 124.

Williamson, J., & Chopin, J. (1980). Adverse reactions to prescribed drugs in the elderly: A multicentre investigation. *Age and Aging, 9,* 73-80.

SECTION II

FUNCTIONAL HEALTH PATTERNS

CHAPTER 4

HEALTH PERCEPTION-
HEALTH MANAGEMENT
FUNCTIONAL HEALTH PATTERN

The maintenance of health becomes more difficult in later life. Additional preventive health practices must be adopted to compensate for increased risks to health associated with organ dysfunction and decline. Bodily changes can alter norms, resulting in the independent identification of problems becoming a greater challenge. The stresses associated with retirement, widowhood, reduced income, and feeling more vulnerable and out of place in a youth-oriented society can weaken reserves and reduce motivation to engage in sound health practices. The misbelief that health deviations are expected, normal consequences of growing old may cause the older person to accept and live with conditions that could be corrected or improved.

The high prevalence of chronic conditions presents another challenge to health maintenance in old age. It is the rare older adult who is free from chronic illness; more typically, the possession of several chronic illnesses is the norm. When one lives with an illness on a chronic basis, health assumes a different meaning. Rather than freedom from disease or a state of physical, emotional or social well-being, a positive health state to a chronically ill person may be judged as being able to move fingers sufficiently to feed oneself, having ample energy to walk three blocks instead of just one, or being less lightheaded from medication. Management of chronic illness can be a large hurdle to overcome. New knowledge and skills may need to be gained. Daily life may be modified due to limitations and care requirements imposed by the illness. The expense of medications and visits to the health care provider can create a financial burden. Leisure activities and social contacts may shrink. Health, a condition frequently taken for granted during earlier years, gradually develops into a significant concern and potentially a major obstacle to a satisfying and normal life-style.

51

GENERIC CARE PLAN FOR THE NURSING DIAGNOSIS
ALTERATION IN HEALTH MAINTENANCE

1. General Information

Alteration in health management is the inability to identify, manage, and/
or seek out help to maintain health. The individual is at risk because of
inadequate preventive measures or an unhealthy life-style.

a. Etiology
  – Alterations in communication skills
  – Perceptual or cognitive impairment
  – Lack of finances
  – Lack of motor skills
  – Unachieved developmental tasks
  – Changing support systems
  – Loss of independence
  – Lack of knowledge
  – Poor learning skills
  – Forced change (e.g., relocation)
  – Inadequate health practices
  – Religious, cultural, and health beliefs
  – Crisis situation
  – Substance abuse

b. Clinical Manifestations
  – History of lack of health-seeking behavior
  – Lack of equipment, finances, personal support
  – Inability to take responsibility for meeting health needs
  – Lack of knowledge regarding health practices
  – Lack of access to health care services

c. Multidisciplinary Approaches
  – Rehabilitation: speech, OT, PT
  – Substance abuse therapy
  – Social service

2. Nursing Process

a. Assessment
  – Progressive illness or a long-term health problem
  – Recent changes in life-style

- Knowledge of resources, use of services
- Level of dependence
- Ability to meet health needs
- Knowledge and skills about health maintenance
- Ability to perform ADL
- Existing health status
- Communication and motor skills
- Income, expenses
- Support systems

b. Goal
Patient's health will be maintained or reestablished at an adequate or improved level.

c. Interventions
- Provide health counseling about home safety, grieving, nutritional changes, sensory changes, and alterations in bowel and bladder habits.
- Encourage good oral hygiene and dental check ups every 6-12 months.
- Recommend physical exam at least every two years.
- Teach self-breast exam to females, and testicle self-exam to males to be done once a month (linking this with a monthly event, such as the day social security checks arrive, is helpful).
- Identify self-care deficits and develop a plan of care with patient (see Chapter 7, Self-care Deficit).
- Listen to the concerns and questions of the patient and family.
- Teach stress management skills.
- Refer as needed to legal services, homemaker, meals-on-wheels, etc.
- Arrange for someone to check on the patient on a regular basis.

d. Evaluation
- Patient's health is reestablished/maintained.
- Patient demonstrates improved coping to meet health needs.

e. Possible Related Nursing Diagnoses
Alteration in thought processes
Impaired communication
Ineffective individual coping
Knowledge deficit
Potential for injury
Self-care deficit

GENERIC CARE PLAN FOR THE NURSING DIAGNOSIS
NONCOMPLIANCE

1. General Information

Noncompliance is personal behavior that deviates from health-related advice given by health care professionals.

a. Etiology
- Physical or mental deficits
- Lack of or insufficient support system
- Insufficient finances
- Insufficient knowledge
- Lack of motivation
- Complex care demands

b. Clinical Manifestations
- No improvement or worsening of health status
- Missed appointments with provider
- Failure to adhere to prescribed diets, drug regimens
- Not obtaining prescriptions or supplies
- Continuance of nonhealthful practices (e.g., smoking, drinking)

c. Multidisciplinary Approaches
- Correct or improve deficits that impede self-care (e.g., pain control, fluid and electrolyte stabilization)
- Social services

2. Nursing Process

a. Assessment
- General health and functional status
- Cognitive function
- Support system
- Knowledge base
- Motivation
- Available resources

b. Goal
Patient's ability to participate in self-care and health practices will improve or an alternative to compensate for deficits will be developed.

c. **Interventions**
- Assist patient in finding means to reduce causative factor, e.g.
  - obtain financial aid
  - arrange for transportation
  - modify environment
  - obtain assistive devices, eyeglasses, hearing aid, walkers
  - teach stress reduction and management techniques.
- Provide counseling and education regarding care requirements, reinforce significance of adhering to care plan.
- Encourage patient to express feelings and concerns.

d. **Evaluation**
- Patient
  - has obstacles to compliance removed or reduced.
  - adheres to care plan.
- Patient's health status improves.

e. **Possible Related Nursing Diagnoses**
Alteration in health maintenance
Anxiety
Disturbance in self-concept
Knowledge deficit
Self-care deficit
Sensory-perceptual alterations

GENERIC CARE PLAN FOR THE NURSING DIAGNOSIS
POTENTIAL FOR INJURY

1. General Information

Potential for injury is a state in which an individual is at risk for accidental injury or trauma because of perceptual or physiologic deficit or lack of awareness, or maturational age.

a. **Etiology**
- Altered mobility
- Impaired sensory function (sight, hearing, tactile sensation)
- Altered cerebral circulatory function
- Pain and fatigue
- Faulty judgment
- Poor coordination and weakness
- Lack of safety education and precautions
- Emotional difficulties
- Altered cognitive function

– Household, automobile, and fire hazards
  • unsafe walkways
  • faulty electric wires
  • throw rugs, slippery or wet floors
  • mechanically unsafe vehicle
  • smoking in bed
  • clutter
  • gas leaks
– Unfamiliar setting (hospital, nursing home)
– Inattentive or abusive caretaker
– Improper use of aids (canes, crutches, walkers, wheelchairs)
– Inappropriate use of hot water bottles, heating pads, sitz baths, heat lamps, enemas, douches
– Inadequate protection from potential sources of burns (particularly significant when patient is mentally impaired)
– Failure to use side rails
– Poor transfer and lifting techniques
– Inadequate protection of confused, sedated, weak, dizzy or visually impaired patient
– Defective or contaminated supplies (e.g., broken wheelchairs, bed with electrical problems)
– Allowing patient to use unapproved appliances
– Loss or damage to eyeglasses, dentures, jewelry
– Delayed response to emergency, injury or complication (e.g., not getting limb x-rayed after fall)
– Inappropriate delegation: allowing unskilled or unapproved person (student, new employee, family member) to perform procedure

b. Clinical Manifestations
– History of accidents
– Motor and sensory deficits
– Lack of knowledge of environmental hazards and safety precautions
– Evidence of environmental hazards (e.g., throw rugs, no hand grips)
– Evidence of physical injury (e.g., bruises, limp, burns)
– Evidence of psychologic injury (e.g., withdrawal, behavior changes)

c. Multidisciplinary Approaches
– Improve cerebral circulation (e.g., blood pressure adjustment)
– Control pain
– Refer for, as necessary, eyeglasses, hearing aids, physical therapy
– Address causative or contributory factor
  • refer to PT, ophthalmologist, audiologist, social worker
  • adjust medication

2. Nursing Process

a. Assessment
- Physical capabilities (mobility, energy, strength)
- Cognitive function, mental status
- Competency of care giver
- Sensory deficits
- Self-care capacities
- Environmental safety
- Knowledge

b. Goal
Patient will be free from injury.

c. Interventions
- Increase patient's ability to protect self by
  - obtaining eyeglasses, hearing aids, canes, walkers
  - improving general health status
  - educating and counseling as necessary
  - orienting to new surroundings
  - supporting treatment plan to improve underlying problem.
- Provide supervision for individual with insufficient cognitive function to protect self.
- Assist with relocation if current living arrangements are hazardous.
- Instruct in safe transfer, ambulation techniques
- Counsel in safe medication use (recognition of side effects, special precautions).
- Remove hazards from environment
  - arrange for correction of electrical, plumbing, heating, appliance problems
  - arrange for homemaker through social service or private agency
  - assist in obtaining grab bars in tubs, handrails
  - assure water heater temperature is not excessive.
- Educate patient in prevention of accidents, emergency measures when accidents do occur.

d. Evaluation
- Patient
  - identifies and protects self against injury.
  - compensates for deficits in self care abilities.
  - experiences no injury.
  - expresses ways to minimize risks and manage emergencies.

e. Possible Related Nursing Diagnoses
Alteration in comfort: pain
Alteration in thought processes

Anxiety
Impaired home maintenance management
Impaired physical mobility
Knowledge deficit
Potential for injury: poisoning
Self-care deficit
Sensory-perceptual alterations

Selected Health Problems Frequently Associated with the Nursing Diagnosis POTENTIAL FOR INJURY
Elderly Abuse

a. Discussion
Elderly abuse occurs to over one million older adults. This number may be low due to the reluctance of victims to report abuse. The gradual build-up of frustration and irritation with the older person frequently results in verbal abuse and negligence rather than physical violence.

b. Etiology
- Care giver
  • frustrated, irritated
  • careless, hurried
  • overstressed, fatigued
  • hostile
- Older person
  • demented, confused
  • demanding
  • frail
  • incontinent
  • helpless, hostile

c. Clinical Manifestations
- Inflicting pain or injury
  • hitting, striking
  • shaking
  • burning or other means
- Unreasonable confinement or restraints
- Stealing personal possessions
- Mismanagement of finances and assests
- Withholding food, care, medications, or services
- Taking sexual advantage
- Administration of inappropriate drugs
- Causing mental or emotional discomfort

d. Multidisciplinary Approaches
- Home health, social service assessment
- Realistic determination of family's capacity to fulfill care-giver responsibilities

Additional Nursing Care That Can Be Incorporated into the Generic Care Plan

- Explore unexplained injuries or subtle indications of mistreatment to help identify potential abuse.
- Remember that most abuse is inflicted by persons closest to the patient (e.g., spouse, child, or direct care giver).
- Report all actual or suspected abuse to the appropriate official agency; don't worry about repercussions; there is usually immunity for parties reporting abuse.
- Realize that it may be wiser to suspect abuse, investigate and find the charge was incorrect than to ignore clues and have the patient incur further injury.

GENERIC CARE PLAN FOR THE NURSING DIAGNOSIS
POTENTIAL FOR INJURY: POISONING

1. General Information

Potential for poisoning is a state wherein the patient has accentuated risk of accidental exposure to or ingestion of drugs or dangerous products in doses sufficient to cause harm.

a. Etiology
- Impaired sensory function (vision, smell)
- Confusion
- Improper use of medications
  - wrong medication or dosage
  - wrong route (e.g., ingestion of a topical drug)
  - improper procedure
- Lack of knowledge (interactions, special precautions)

b. Clinical Manifestations
- Lack of safety or drug education
- Lack of proper precautions
- Cognitive difficulties
- Large variety of drugs
- Dangerous products stored near confused person
- Availability of illicit drugs
- Unprotected contact with heavy metals or chemicals

- Exposure to atmospheric pollutants
- Inability to differentiate various tastes, odors

c. **Multidisciplinary Approaches**
- Selective prescription of medications
- Improvement of conditions interfering with safe drug use (e.g., pain control, prosthesis)

2. Nursing Process

a. **Assessment**
- Mental status
- Physical health, functional capacity, sensory function
- Knowledge of medications
- Types of prescription and nonprescription medications including dosage, frequency of dosage
- Environment
- Support systems

b. **Goal**
Patient will protect self or be protected from accidental poisoning.

c. **Interventions**
- Assure medications are prescribed only when absolutely necessary; use nonpharmacologic alternatives when possible.
- Educate patient and care givers in safe use of medications (purpose, dosage, route, interactions, side effects); advise against self-prescription.
- Because of adverse effects of all drugs, monitor patient to ensure prompt recognition of problems.
- For cognitively impaired patients, safeguard environment to prevent injury (e.g., lock up medications and noningestible substances, supervise activities, observe closely).
- Administer medications appropriately (correct dosage, route, patient).
- Assure hazardous substances are clearly labelled.
- Caution patient not to put drugs or potentially poisonous substances into different containers.

d. **Evaluation**
- Patient
  - experiences no signs of adverse reaction to prescription medications.
  - uses nonprescription drugs as directed.
  - environmental risks are removed or decreased.

e. **Possible Related Nursing Diagnoses**
    Alteration in comfort: pain
    Alteration in health maintenance
    Alteration in thought processes
    Impaired physical mobility
    Ineffective individual coping
    Knowledge deficit
    Noncompliance
    Self-care deficit
    Sensory-perceptual alterations

GENERIC CARE PLAN FOR THE NURSING DIAGNOSIS
POTENTIAL FOR INFECTION

1. General Information

The elderly are more prone to develop infections. Age reduces efficiency of antibody production and there is a greater prevalence of disease conditions promoting bacterial growth (e.g., diabetes, cancer). A decrease in the endocrine system's functioning affects not only the elderly's metabolic rate but lends them more vulnerable to infections and diseases.
Endocrine system changes seen in the elderly include
  – marked decrease in ability to fight disease
  – increase in autoimmune properties
  – increased susceptibility to disease, especially chronic disease
  – decrease in glucose tolerance
  – reduced production of gonadal hormones
  – decreased production of thyroid stimulating hormone (TSH) and thyroid hormone
As the aged lung becomes more rigid there are reduced respirations and cough efficiency, decreased ability to remove secretions, and less sensitive pharyngeal reflexes. The combination of reduced capacity to cough and deep breathe and impaired mobility render the geriatric patient vulnerable to respiratory infections.
Urinary tract infections in women in most cases are caused by *E. coli* associated with poor hygiene. In men, most cases are due to *P. vulgaris* associated with prostatic disease. Clogged catheters, urinary retention, and diabetes (excess urinary protein, glucose promote bacterial growth) also contribute to this common problem in the geriatric patient.
Vaginitis can arise from age-related changes in the vaginal canal such as increased alkalinity of vaginal secretions.

a. **Etiology**
    – Altered antigen-antibody reaction
    – Respiratory changes
    – Genitourinary changes
    – Skin fragility

- Immobility, disability
- Catheter use
- Malnutrition
- Immunosuppressive or radiation therapy
- Poor hygiene

b. Clinical Manifestations
- Elevated temperature, night sweats
- Aches and pain
- Cough, sputum
- Increased respiratory rate
- Fatigue and malaise
- Loss of appetite
- Burning, urgency (urination)
- Itching, discharge (vaginitis)
- Lesions, ulcerated or reddened skin
- Stiff, swollen joints

c. Medical Management
- Antibiotics (see Table 4.1)
- Possible isolation

Table 4.1   Review of Selected Antibiotics

Antibiotic	Possible Adverse Effects	Nursing Implications
Ampicillin Carbenicillin	Rash, fever or chills, diarrhea, nausea, vomiting, irritations of mouth or tongue	Question patient regarding past allergic reaction to penicillin; even if no previous history, observe carefully for reaction; reduced dosages may be required for patients with altered liver or renal function. Instruct patients taking ampicillin –keep taking for number of days specified even if symptoms subside –call physician if side effects develop –administer 3 hours before or after meals –don't save drug and use for future infections in self or family. If administered orally, do not administer 3 hours before or after meals (prevents absorption problems). If administered intravenously, change site every 48 hours, observe carefully (high risk of vein irritation). Monitor serum potassium.

Table 4.1   Review of Selected Antibiotics (continued)

Antibiotic	Possible Adverse Effects	Nursing Implications
Cephaclor	Rash, headache, drowsiness, dizziness, nausea, vomiting, indigestion, diarrhea, abdominal cramping, irritation of mouth or tongue	Contraindicated in paitents with history of allergic reaction to any cephalosporin. Since cephalosporins are nephrotoxic, use with care in persons with impaired renal function. Persons sensitive to penicillin will have greater likelihood of allergic reaction to cephalosporins. May be administered with meals. More expensive than any antibiotics.
Doxycycline	Rash, anorexia, nausea, vomiting, diarrhea, irritation of mouth or tongue	Do not expose to light or heat. Administer with meals or milk. High risk of thrombophlebitis with IV administration. Alters results of Clinitest and similar urine tests.
Erythromycin	Rash, hives, nausea, vomiting, diarrhea, liver damage with long-term use	Erythromycin estolate is contraindicated in persons with impaired liver function; can cause hepatotoxicity. Coated tablets can be taken with meals, otherwise take 2 hours before or after eating. Tablets should be followed by at least 8 oz water; should not be administered with juices.
Kanamycin	Ototoxicity (tinnitus, vertigo, headache, nausea, vomiting, hearing loss)	Use with extreme caution in elderly due to nephrotoxicity. Monitor renal function closely (e.g., I&O, weight, BUN). Encourage good fluid intake to help reduce the concentration of kanamycin in kidney tissue. Obtain baseline audiometric reading and reevaluate periodically throughout therapy. Toxic effects more likely when blood level exceeds 30 mcg/ml.
Nitrofurantoin	Dyspnea, coughing, asthmatic attacks, other respiratory problems	Contraindicated in persons with impaired kidney function. Administer with food or milk. Urine may become dark or brown (not significant); note I&O. Discontinue at the first sign of respiratory reaction. Can cause false glycosurias with Clinitest. May take 1–2 weeks of therapy for noticeable response; evaluate

(continued)

Table 4.1 Review of Selected Antibiotics (continued)

Antibiotic	Possible Adverse Effects	Nursing Implications
		urine specimens for culture and sensitivity periodically during therapy. Store in a dark, nonmetallic container.
Sulfisoxazole	Rashes, anorexia, abdominal pain, irritation of mouth, tinnitus, tingling of extremities, acute mental or behavioral disturbance; hemolytic anemia, bone marrow depression, hepatitis and kidney damage (hemolytic anemia can occur when sulfisoxazole is taken with isoniazid)	Contraindicated in persons with a history of allergic reaction to any sulfonamide ("sulfa" drug); used with caution in persons with liver or kidney disease, history of bronchial asthma, or allergies. Take with a full glass of water; encourage good fluid intake to prevent crystals from forming in urine. Monitor I&O. Urine may become dark or brown—not significant. Initiate vitamin C replacement therapy only *after* sulfisoxazole is discontinued (vitamin C administered during therapy will make the urine more acidic, contributing to crystal formation).

Interactions
Ampicillin and Carbenicillin
• effects decreased by antacids, chloramphenicol, erythromycin, tetracycline.
Cephaclor
• effects increased by probenecid.
Doxycycline
• absorption decreased when administered with aluminum, calcium- or magnesium-based laxatives, antacids, iron preparations, phenobartectal, alcohol.
Erythromycin
• penicillins will antagonize effects of erythromycin and vice versa; do not give penicillin within 2 hours of erythromycin.
Nitrofurantoin
• effects increased by probenecid.
• effects decreased by phenobarbital.
Sulfisoxazole
• Increases effects of alcohol, oral anticoagulants, oral antidiabetic agents, methotrexate, phenytoin.
• decreases effects of penicillin.
• effects increased by aspirin, oxyphenbutazone, phenylbutazone, probenecid, promethazine, sulfinpyrazone, trimethoprim.
• effects decreased by paraldehyde, para-aminosalicylic acid.

2. Nursing Process

a. Assessment
   — Signs and symptoms of infections
   — High-risk factors such as fragility, immobility, chronic disease
   — Changes in behavior

b. **Goals**
Patient
 − will be free from infection.
 − will have potential hazards minimized to prevent recurrence.

c. **Interventions**
 − Encourage good nutrition by emphasizing adequate protein and vitamins.
 − Increase fluids (if not contraindicated) to lessen chance of dehydration and electrolyte imbalance.
 − Adhere to proper handwashing and hygienic practices, aseptic technique where applicable.
 − Offer cranberry and prune juices to maintain acid urine, which reduces bacterial growth in urine.
 − Don't use catheters unless absolutely essential as most people develop urinary tract infections within one week of catheterization.
 − Handle and store food safely.
 − Prevent skin breakdown by promoting good skin care (see Skin Integrity).
 − Isolate patients who have communicable diseases and screen visitors.
 − Follow aseptic technique, isolation procedure if indicated.
 − Be alert to unusual signs and symptoms; subnormal body temperature may distort manifestation of fever and pain may be referred.
 − Offer periodic tuberculosis screening for high-risk elderly who are institutionalized, exposed to large groups, or living in poor conditions.
 − Maintain clean environment and handle wastes carefully.
 − Provide good oral hygiene.
 − Keep both patient and clothing and linens dry.
 − Offer massages, cold compresses for headache.
 − Conserve energy.
 − Administer antibiotics and analgesics as ordered; note precautions and interactions (see Tables 4.1 and 8.5).
 − Be aware of the various antibiotics that could be used and organisms for which they are effective; assure that the proper antibiotic is being used for the infection being treated.
 − Observe for adverse reactions: the elderly are more sensitive to antibiotics; monitor closely.
 − Note signs of new infections (e.g., moniliasis, diarrhea); superinfections can develop from long-term use of antibiotics.
 − Remember that elderly persons often respond more slowly to antibiotic therapy.

d. **Evaluation**
 − Patient's infection is controlled and not spread to others.
 − Patient
   • has symptomatic relief.
   • is free from complications of drug therapy.

e. Possible Related Nursing Diagnoses

Activity intolerance
Alteration in comfort
Alteration in nutrition: less than body requirements
Alteration in respiratory function
Fluid volume deficit
Impairment of skin integrity
Potential for infection to others

References

Barbieri, E. (1983). Patient falls are not patient accidents. *Journal of Gerontological Nursing, 9*(3), 165-172.

Beck C., & Phillips, L. (1982). Abuse of the elderly. *Journal of Gerontological Nursing, 8*(2), 22-26.

Brody, S., & Persily, N. (1984). *Hospitals and the aged. The new old market.* Rockville, MD: Aspen Systems Corp.

Chipman, C., & Sarano, G. (1984). Falls and their consequences. In A. Schwartz, G. Bosker, & J. Grigsby (Eds.), *Geriatric emergencies.* Bowie, MD: Brady.

Cooper, S. (1981). Common concern: Accidents and older adults. *Geriatric Nursing, 2*(4), 289-290.

Gleckman, R., & Gantz, N. (Eds.). *Infections in the elderly.* Boston: Little, Brown.

Hayter, J. (1980). Hypothermia/hyperthermia in older persons. *Journal of Gerontological Nursing, 6*(2), 65-68.

Higgins, P. (1983). Can 98.6 be a fever in disguise? *Geriatric Nursing, 4*(2), 101-102.

Kalchthaler, T., Bascon, R., & Quintos, V. (1978). Falls in the institutionalized elderly. *Journal of the American Geriatrics Society, 26*(9), 424-428.

Kauffman, C., & Jones, P. (1984). Diagnosing fever of unknown origin in older patients. *Geriatrics, 39*(2), 46-54.

King, P. (1980). Foot problems and their assessment. *Geriatric Nursing, 1*, 182.

Koin, D. (1984). Abuse and neglect in the aged. In G. Schwartz, C. Bosker, & J. Grigsley (Eds.), *Geriatric emergencies.* Bowie, MD: Brady.

Kolanowski, A., & Gunther, L. (1981). Hypothermia in the elderly. *Geriatric Nursing, 2*(5), 362-365.

Kustaborder, M., & Rigney, M. (1983). Interventions for safety. *Journal of Gerontological Nursing, 9*(3), 185-193.

Lawton, M. (1983). Environment and other determinents of well being in older people. *Gerontologist, 23*(4), 349-357.

Lonnerblad, L. (1984). Exercises to promote independent living in older patients. *Geriatrics, 39*(2), 93-101.

Mitchell, R. (1984). Falls in the elderly. *Nursing Times, 80*(2), 51-3.

Overstall, P. (1980). Prevention of falls in the elderly. *Journal of the American Geriatrics Society, 28*(11), 481-483.

Palmer, M. (1982). Assisting the older woman with cosmetics. *Journal of Gerotological Nursing, 8*, 340.

Riffle, K. (1982). Falls: Kinds, causes and prevention. *Geriatric Nursing, 3*(3), 165-169.

Roberts, B., & Fitzpatrick, J. (1983). Improving balance: Therapy of movement. *Journal of Gerontological Nursing, 9*(3), 150-156.

Rowe, J., & Besdine, R. (Eds.). (1982). *Health and disease in old age.* Boston: Little, Brown.

Rubenstein, L., & Robbins, A. (1984). Falls in the elderly: Clinical perspective. *Geriatrics, 39*(4), 67-78.

Saddington, N. (1983). Winter of discontent? . . . Hypothermia is only one of many problems the elderly face. *Nursing Times, 79*(43), 10-11.

Smith, I. (1983). Infectious disease problems in the elderly. In W. Reichel (Ed.), *Clinical aspects of aging* (2nd ed.). Baltimore: Williams & Wilkins.

Thatcher, R. (1983). 98.6° F.—What is normal? *Journal of Gerontological Nursing, 9*(1), 22-27.

CHAPTER 5

NUTRITIONAL-METABOLIC
FUNCTIONAL HEALTH PATTERN

Proper diet is especially important for older persons to promote optimal physical and mental function, increase resistance to disease, and reduce secondary problems associated with existing chronic illnesses. Receiving adequate nutrients can become a major concern of the elderly because of changes in the digestive system and life-long poor dietary practices. A slower metabolic rate results in a reduced energy expenditure and lower calorie requirements, which should be individually determined based on patient's height, weight, health, and activity.

Although total body protein decreases with age, protein requirements do not significantly change (males: 56 gm/day, females: 46 gm/day). Carbohydrates make up more than one-half the average diet. Controversy surrounds the issue of fat consumption. Studies indicate that high saturated fat diets promote higher cholesterol levels and atherosclerotic disease. Some fats are necessary to enhance metabolism of the fat-soluble vitamins A, D, E, and K.

Vitamin requirements are consistent throughout the lifespan. Adequate intake can be achieved through ingestion of a well-balanced diet of fruits, vegetables and dairy products, making vitamin supplements unnecessary (see Table 5.1). Vitamin supplements may be indicated in cases of absorption problems, inadequate dietary intake, unusual stress, and healing. Megadoses have no proven benefit and may produce adverse effects, e.g., high doses of vitamin C can exacerbate gout by raising the uric acid level.

A negative calcium balance is normal in older persons and 0.4-0.8 gm/day is needed to compensate for the loss. Regular milk and dairy product intake should be sufficient to satisfy daily calcium needs. The normal requirement for iron is 1-2 mg/day. Red meats, eggs, green vegetables, milk, and iron-fortified bread can provide ample iron intake. Supplements need not be taken unless iron-deficiency anemia is present. Daily requirements of other minerals are obtainable through a normal diet containing seafood, dark green leafy vegetables, dairy products, whole grain breads and cereals.

Fiber (intake: 30-60 gm/day) promotes good elimination and can be obtained through fruits, vegetables, and whole grain breads and cereals. Unless contraindicated, between 2500-3000 cc of fluid should be consumed each day.

There are many causes of altered nutrition in the elderly. Many of the physical, emotional, and social problems of the elderly, in addition to sensory changes, can lead to a profound impairment in food intake that can seriously threaten their health and well-being.

Physiologic Factors

- Decreased secretion of enzymes; indigestion common
- Decreased absorption of nutrients and minerals
- Reduced motility of stomach; slowing of peristalsis
- Additional problems caused by problems with teeth and dentures (e.g., receding gums, ill-fitting dentures, periodontal disease, missing teeth)
- Decrease in flow of saliva
- Decreased ability to detect pleasant odors and taste sweet and salty foods due to a decline in the number of taste buds on the tongue

Psychosocial Factors

- Decreased access to proper foods due to poverty
- Misinformation about dietary needs and nutritional value of foods
- Less money to purchase proper foods
- Sociocultural background, beliefs, attitudes, personal preferences
- Reduction in exercise
- Physical/mental incapacity to prepare meals
- Diet altered through diseases such as alcoholism
- Loneliness and depression of eating alone

Table 5.1 Recommended Daily Vitamin Intake for Persons Over Age 65

Vitamin	Recommended Dose/Day (Female/Male)
A	4,500–5,000 International Units (IU)
B Complex	
Thiamine (B_1)	1.0–1.1 mg/1.3–1.5 mg
Riboflavin (B_2)	1.3–1.5 mg/1.3–1.7 mg
Niacin (B_3)	12–16 mg/14–20 mg
Pyridoxine (B_6)	1.4–2 mg
Cobalamin (B_{12})	5–6 mcg
Folic Acid	0.4 mg
Biotin	0.1–0.2 mg
Pantothenic Acid	4–7 mg
C	40–55 mg/40–60 mg
D	400 IU
E	20–25 IU/20–30 IU
K	0.3–15 mg/kg of body weight

   – Lack of energy and interest in food
   – Lack of cooking facilities

GENERIC CARE PLAN FOR THE NURSING DIAGNOSIS
ALTERATION IN NUTRITION: LESS THAN BODY REQUIREMENTS

1. General Information

Occurs when there is an insufficient intake of nutrients to meet metabolic needs.

a. Etiology
– Knowledge deficit about minimum daily requirements
– Pain with mastication, poor condition of teeth, dentures
– Altered taste sensation
– Anorexia
– Emotional stress
– Social isolation
– Inability to procure or prepare food
– Financial limitations
– Inability to ingest or digest food or absorb nutrients
– Sore, inflamed buccal cavity

b. Clinical Manifestations
– 20% or more under ideal body weight
– Triceps skin fold, mid-arm circumference less than 60% of standard measurement
– Reported inadequate food intake
– Muscle weakness and tenderness, fatigue
– Mental irritability or confusion
– Evidence of lack of food intake
– Aversion to eating
– Diarrhea, hyperactive bowel sounds
– Poor skin turgor, pallor

c. Multidisciplinary Approaches
– Identify and correct underlying problems, e.g.
   • remove loose or diseased teeth
   • treat periodontal disease
   • prescribe appetite stimulants
   • psychiatric interventions
   • diagnostic tests for CA, digitalis toxicity, renal insufficienty, etc.
– Secure nutritional resources (e.g., Meals-on-Wheels)

2. Nursing Process

a. Assessment
- Precise weight of patient, using the same scale, same clothes, and weigh at same time of day
- Ability to chew, swallow, taste; denture fit, status of oral cavity
- Triceps skinfold thickness
- Laboratory analysis of blood, serum vitamin and electrolyte levels
- Detailed diet history
  - usual eating habits (be specific, e.g., "What is the first thing you eat each day and when do you eat it?" "How many spoons of sugar do you add to your coffee?")
  - food likes, dislikes, and restrictions
  - use of alcohol and drugs (prescription and nonprescription), use of antacids, laxatives, diuretics
  - food intolerances and preferences
- Need for diary of total daily caloric intake, times and patterns of eating
- Psychologic factors and cultural preferences; body image and patient's view of self
- Ability to afford, shop for, prepare, and store food
- Existing health problems
- Recent losses and stresses

b. Goal
Patient will ingest a diet that satisfies some preferences and conforms to prescribed restrictions yet contains all needed nutrients.

c. Interventions
- Use assessment information to plan meals; avoid foods that cause intolerance; offer favored, culturally important foods.
- Modify diet as necessary: dietary supplements, increase protein, CHO, calories; offer frequent small meals, soft foods, appetite stimulants (e.g., small amount of wine).
- Maximize the nutrient content of each calorie ingested (e.g., a doughnut and a glass of milk may both have the same amount of calories, but the milk will offer 4 times the amount of protein and minerals).
- Judge carbohydrate intake in relation to caloric needs, reduce intake of simple carbohydrates (e.g., sugar) and replace with complex carbohydrates (e.g., cereals, breads).
- Enhance food by using flavoring (lemon, herbs, salt); promote a pleasant and relaxing atmosphere for eating with other people if possible.
- Prevent early satiety by limiting fiber/bulk and limit fluids 1 hour prior to meals.
- Teach patient importance of balanced diet and need for a consistent intake of nutrients to reach and maintain ideal weight.

- Expect the time for eating and digestion to be increased; do not rush the patient—feed slowly.
- Caution patient against factors that can interfere with absorption of nutrients (e.g., alcohol and tobacco).
- Be alert to food-drug interactions (e.g., liver, spinach, turnip greens, cabbage, and broccoli can interfere with the effectiveness of oral anticoagulants; antacids can reduce the potency of oral antibiotics, digoxin, oral anticoagulants, and salicylates).
- Identify and act early on subtle signs of nutritional problems (see Table 5.2).

Table 5.2 Signs of Nutritional Problems

Nutritional Problem	Signs and Symptoms
Vitamin A deficiency	Dry skin Persistent "goose bumps" Night blindness
Vitamin B_6 deficiency	Red, scaly skin (all body parts) Burning feet Hypochromic anemia Depression Confusion
Vitamin B_{12} deficiency	Weakness, pallor Dyspnea Sore tongue or mouth Anorexia Burning sensation in limbs Hypotension; tachycardia Ataxia
Vitamin C deficiency	Purpura Swollen, bleeding gums (except in the edentulous)
Vitamin D deficiency	Bone pain and tenderness Frequent or unexplained fractures
Vitamin K deficiency (hypoprothrombinemia)	Purpura
Iron deficiency	Pallor Weakness Fatigue
Magnesium deficiency	Vertigo Seizures Muscle weakness Tremors Depression; irritability
Niacin deficiency (Pellagra)	Sore mouth Brownish pigmentation of skin exposed to light Dermatitis Diarrhea Depression Confusion

(continued)

Table 5.2   Signs of Nutritional Problems (continued)

Nutritional Problem	Signs and Symptoms
Phosphate deficiency	Fatigue, malaise Muscle weakness Bone pain
Potassium deficiency	Weakness Drowsiness Nausea Vomiting
Riboflavin deficiency	Red, scaly skin, folds around eyes and between nose and corners of mouth Fissures in corner of mouth Smooth, purple and sore tongue Genital dermatitis
Zinc deficiency	Dermatitis, primarily in periphery of limbs Decreased taste sensation Delayed wound healing
Hyperglycemia	Fungus infection Recurrent boils
Hyperuricemia	Gout

- Be aware of dietary restrictions/demands associated with specific diseases; instruct patient in terms of "eating healthy" rather than a diet that connotes a restriction.
- Unless contraindicated, occasionally give candy to satisfy craving for sweets that is common in the aged.
- Assist patient to modify present habits rather than force major changes in habits because older people find it difficult to change lifelong patterns of eating.
- Encourage patient to discuss feelings of deprivation and how to plan for an occasional treat within diet.

d. Evaluation
- Patient
  • maintains adequate nutritional intake.
  • gains/maintains weight.
  • demonstrates necessary changes in eating patterns, food quality and quantity.
- Patient's laboratory values are within normal limits.

e. Possible Related Nursing Diagnoses
Alteration in bowel elimination: constipation
Fluid volume deficit
Self-care deficit, feeding
Sensory-perceptual alterations: gustatory and olfactory

Selected Health Problems Frequently Associated with the Nursing Diagnosis ALTERATION IN NUTRITION: LESS THAN BODY REQUIREMENTS

1. Anorexia

a. **Definition**
Anorexia refers to the loss of appetite and lack of interest in food.

b. **Etiology**
   – Physical diseases
      • anemia, cancer
      • chronic obstructive pulmonary disease
   – Emotional illness (depression, anxiety)
   – Life crisis
   – Social isolation
   – Drugs

c. **Clinical Manifestations**
   – No interest in food
   – Reduced food intake
   – Weight loss
   – Fatigue, weakness
   – Mental status alterations

d. **Multidisciplinary Approaches**
   – Vitamins and mineral supplements
   – Psychiatric and social interventions

Additional Nursing Care That Can Be Incorporated into the Generic Care Plan

   – Urge family and friends to prepare special meals that patient is known to like.
   – Provide good oral hygiene before and after meals.
   – Provide meals in pleasant surroundings
      • allow socialization
      • remove bedpans, treatment supplies, and litter
      • serve food in comfortable area.
   – Present food attractively
      • serve at correct temperatures
      • vary colors and textures
      • avoid styrofoam and plastic plates and utensils

- have tablecloth and flowers on table and background music, if possible
- group dining if possible.
— Offer several small rather than a few large servings.

Other Possible Nursing Diagnoses

Ineffective individual coping
Potential for infection

2. Anemia

a. **Definition**
   A condition in which there is a reduced red blood cell count and a subnormal hemoglobin or hematocrit level. It is a common finding in the elderly.

b. **Etiology**
   — *Iron deficiency anemia* may be due to insufficient dietary intake of iron, impaired iron absorption, or excess bleeding.
   — *Pernicious anemia* is caused by impaired absorption of vitamin B_{12} or stomach cancer.
   — *Aplastic anemia* is a serious form of anemia that has no discernible cause in approximately half of all cases; known etiologies include radiation, drugs (analgesics, diuretics, hypoglycemic agents, antihistamines), or chemicals (insecticides).

c. **Clinical Manifestations**
   — Pallor, fatigue
   — Poor skin turgor
   — Change in mental status
   — Increased cardiac output
   — Palpitations, angina
   — Headache, dizziness
   — Dyspnea
   — Pernicious anemia
     • anorexia
     • smooth red tongue
     • gastrointestinal symptoms
     • weight loss
     • indigestion
     • recurring diarrhea and constipation
     • infection
   — Aplastic anemia
     • purpura
     • bleeding

d. Multidisciplinary Approaches
  – Diagnostic studies
    • serum B_{12} analysis
    • gastric analysis
    • Schilling test
    • bone marrow aspiration
  – Oral or injectible iron supplements
  – B_{12} injections
  – Packed cells transfusions
  – Steroids and androgens

Additional Nursing Care That Can Be Incorporated into the Generic Care Plan

  – Increase patient's consumption of iron-rich foods (e.g., green leafy vegetables, meat, fish, poultry, dried fruits, enriched breads and cereals).
  – Encourage vitamin C intake (ascorbic acid promotes iron absorption).
  – Prepare patient for indigestion, change in stool color, and constipation when giving iron supplements.
  – Administer and observe for side effects of steroids and androgens if prescribed.
  – Provide for rest periods between activities and treat ment.
  – Assist with blood transfusions, if ordered; monitor carefully for symptoms of transfusion reaction.

Other Possible Nursing Diagnosis

  Potential for infection

3. Cirrhosis

a. Definition:
  A progressive disease of the liver characterized by tissue scarring primarily affecting persons between ages 40–70 and men nearly twice as frequently as women. It ranks as the ninth leading cause of death in the elderly.

b. Etiology
  – Alcoholism (primary cause)
  – Hepatitis
  – Biliary obstruction

c. Clinical Manifestions
  – Jaundice
  – Dark, rust-colored urine
  – Clay-colored stools

- Portal hypertension
- Bleeding tendencies
- Edema
- Drowsiness
- Confusion
- Reduced resistance to infection

d. Multidisciplinary Approaches
- Diagnostic tests
  - serum alkaline phosphatase, SGOT, prothrombin time
  - hepatic scanning
  - liver biopsy
- Vitamins A, D, K, and B complex, folic acid
- Dietary modification: moderately high protein, high calorie, sodium restricted (if fluid retention present) to 200–500 mg daily; protein often needs to be restricted
- Possible palliative surgery: portocaval shunt
- Alcoholic treatment and counseling

Additional Nursing Care That Can Be Incorporated into the Generic Care Plan

- Maintain bedrest as needed and ordered.
- Offer small meals frequently rather than large ones, encourage use of supplements.
- Emphasize need to eliminate alcohol from diet; offer referrals to alcohol cessation therapy if necessary/desired.
- Be aware of ordered medications that are metabolized in the liver (dosage adjustment or drug change may be necessary).
- Monitor edema, ascites, jaundice.
- Identify early signs of bleeding, abnormalities (e.g., nosebleeds, bleeding gums, unexplained bruises, petechiae).
- Test every stool for occult blood.
- Take vital signs regularly, observe for changes.
- Regularly assess patient's mental status (hepatic coma is a serious complication of this condition).
- Offer regular skin care for cleansing, relief of pruritus.

GENERIC CARE PLAN FOR THE NURSING DIAGNOSIS ALTERATION IN NUTRITION: MORE THAN BODY REQUIREMENTS

1. General Information

a. Etiology
- Diet high in simple and complex carbohydrates
- Reduced activity

 – Depression, boredom
 – Metabolic abnormalities
 – Knowledge deficit regarding nutritional needs

b. **Clinical Manifestations**
 – 20% or more above ideal body weight
 – Documented intake in excess of metabolic requirements
 – Evidence of unbalanced diet (e.g., high in carbohydrates and fat, low in protein)
 – Pattern of sedentary activity either enforced or by choice

c. **Multidisciplinary approaches**
 – Dietary counseling
 – Physical therapy; exercise regimen
 – Increased activity schedule
 – Behavior modification

2. Nursing Process

a. **Assessment**
 – Patient's perceptions of body weight
 – Patient's precise weight, using the same scale, same clothes and weigh at same time of day
 – Weight compared to ideal weight charts
 – Detailed diet history
 – Patterns of eating
 – Previous attempts at weight reduction
 – Physical problems related to weight (e.g., decreased mobility, impaired skin integrity, fatigue, weakness)

b. **Goals**
Patient
 – will regain and maintain ideal body weight ± 10%.
 – will express satisfaction with dietary restrictions and weight adjustment.
Patient's diet will be balanced within caloric restrictions.

c. **Interventions**
 – Determine caloric needs and restrictions.
 – Teach patient and family about potential problems resulting in or from nutritional excess (e.g., disease process, medication side effects, impaired mobility).
 – Provide diet counseling as patient is ready to accept it; include menu planning, identification of behavior that leads to overeating, behavior modification, group therapy, and physical exercise.
 – Facilitate compliance with prescribed diet by providing positive reinforcement.

- Work with patient to develop a regimen to increase activity and decrease calorie consumption (provide opportunity for physical activity, limit snacks).
- Provide emotional support for the family and patient learning new behaviors (specify behaviors, e.g., altered cooking methods, exercise, changed eating habits).

d. Evaluation
- Patient
  - adheres to dietary restrictions.
  - loses weight at a safe rate.
  - establishes a regular activity program.

e. Possible Related Nursing Diagnoses
Disturbance in self-concept
Knowledge deficit
Ineffective individual coping
Potential for injury

Selected Health Problems Frequently Associated with the Nursing Diagnosis ALTERATION IN NUTRITION: MORE THAN BODY REQUIREMENTS

1. Diabetes Mellitus

a. Definition
A chronic, hereditary disease in which an abnormally high blood glucose level exists as a result of insufficient insulin or lack of insulin production. Problems in the metabolism of carbohydrates, protein, and fat occur. It is thought to be the most prevalent metabolic disease among the elderly possibly because of improved diagnostic tools and the fact that greater numbers of people are living longer.

Diabetes first diagnosed at an older age may be controlled with diet alone or with oral hypoglycemic agents. Older patients with longstanding, insulin-dependent diabetes may be suffering some of the long-term risks of this disease, including retinopathy and cardiovascular problems.

Diabetes may be first detected during the investigation of other problems such as orthostatic hypotension, stroke, gastric hypotony, neuropathy, impotence, Dypuytren's contracture, or glaucoma.

It is important to recognize the unreliability of many conventional diabetic testing methods in older patients. Changes with age can allow hyperglycemia without demonstrable glycosuria and negate the clinical significance of glycosuria. Some older diabetics have normal fasting glucose levels but become hyperglycemic following meals. Glucose tolerance testing, using age-adjusted gradients for interpretation, is the most effective means of diabetic diagnosis in the elderly. Hyperglycemia and glyscosuria are not definite indicators of diabetes since research now shows that blood glucose levels rise slightly with normal aging. Age-related changes in renal function may cause glucosuria without hyperglycemia.

b. **Etiology**
   - Total or partial lack of insulin production
   - Physiologic deterioration in glucose tolerance as a result of advanced age

c. **Clinical Manifestations**
   - Fatigue
   - Drowsiness after meals
   - Weight loss
   - Irritability
   - Nocturia
   - Pruritus
   - Slow wound healing
   - Easier development of infections
   - Blurred vision
   - Muscle cramps

d. **Multidisciplinary Approaches**
   - Dietary modification
   - Medications (see Tables 5.3 and 5.4)
     • insulin
     • oral hypoglycemic agents
   - Life-style modifications (e.g., activity, diet, foot care)

Additional Nursing Care That Can Be Incorporated into the Generic Care Plan

   - Prepare the patient in advance for diabetic (glucose tolerance) testing
     • provide a high (at least 150 gm) carbohydrate diet for several days beforehand
     • explain that blood will be drawn at regular intervals (before glucose administration, 1, 2, and 3 hours after administration)
     • be alert to signs of unusual stress, illness, malnutrition, or inactivity prior to testing; report to physician
     • ask every patient being tested about salicylate use; many elderly self-medicate with aspirin to relieve arthritic pain
     • advise the physician if patient is taking medications (e.g., ethacrynic acid, furosemide, estrogen, propranolol, salicylates) that can affect glucose tolerance

- use age-related gradients to interpret test findings (add 10 mg glucose for each decade over age 55 to the first, second, and third hour standard value); make no adjustment to the first (fasting) blood sample
- inform patient that several glucose tolerance tests may be required before diagnosis is confirmed.

Table 5.3 Antidiabetic Drugs

Example	Common Side Effects	Nursing Implications
Injectable Insulin Oral hypoglycemic agents Tolbutamide Chlorpropamide Tolazamide	Insulin allergy: local redness, swelling, pain and nodule development at injection site Insulin lipodystrophy: atrophy and hypertrophy at injection site Increased sensitivity to sunlight Hypoglycemia (insulin shock) —confusion, disorientation —behavioral changes —anxiety —chills —perspiration —pallor —drowsiness —headache —nausea —weakness —tachycardia Hyperglycemia (ketoacidosis) —thirst —anorexia —vomiting —hot, flushed appearance —listlessness, drowsiness —sweet, fruity breath —decreased blood pressure	Begin with low insulin dosage; gradually increase until desired effect achieved with fewest side effects (dosage is determined by weight). Teach patient (and care givers) to recognize signs of hypo- and hyperglycemia. Be alert to unique signs of diabetic conditions in the elderly (e.g., confusion, slurred speech) as first indications of hypoglycemia. Consult physician about dosage adjustment if indicated by NPO status, surgery, or change in diet, activity schedule. Have patient wear bracelet or other identifying device to indicate diabetic status.

Interactions: Insulin
Increases effect of alcohol, oral anticoagulants, isoniazid, MAO inhibitors, phenylbutazone, salicylates (large dosages), sulfinpyrazine.
Decreases effect of chlorpromazine, cortisonelike drugs, furosemide, phenytoin, thiazide diuretics, thyroid preparations.

- Instruct patient in recognition of signs and symptoms of hyperglycemia and hypoglycemia (see Table 5.3).
- Observe for signs of infection, particularly fungal and urinary tract infection (see Chapter 6, Urinary Tract Infections).
- Be alert to situations that can impact antidiabetic management (e.g., change in diet, activity, surgery, stressful situations, new medication).
- Teach proper dietary practices
  - important not to miss meals
  - change in activity alters food and medication requirement
  - reduce and maintain weight at an appropriate level
  - use guides and lists (available from nutritionists) to identify nutritive content of various foods.
- Teach proper foot care by having patient regularly exercise feet; inspect for abnormalities, discolorations, skin breakdown, change in temperature (see Table 5.5).
- Advise patient to tell all health care providers with whom s/he comes in contact about diabetic condition.
- Instruct patient to wear an ID bracelet and carry identification card in wallet that describes condition.
- Label patient's medical records.
- Administer antidiabetic medications as prescribed
  - begin with low dose and gradually increase until desired effect is achieved (see Table 5.4).
  - know that dosage is determined by weight and activity.
  - consult physician about need for dosage adjustment related to surgery, NPO status, change in diet and/or activity.
  - review all medications administered for potential interactions (see Table 5.3).
- Educate patient on self-injection if required
  - obtain special syringes/appliance to compensate for poor eyesight, arthritic joints, or other factors that could complicate injection; American Diabetes Association, occupational therapists, or rehabilitation staff may be of assistance.
  - advise about proper storage (e.g., do not keep insulin unrefrigerated more than seven days).

Table 5.4 Insulin Action and Duration

Type	Action Onset	Peak	Duration
Regular	½–1 hour	2–3 hours	5–7 hours
Semilente	½–1 hour	5–8 hours	12–16 hours
Globin Zinc	1–2 hours	6–12 hours	18–24 hours
NPH	1–3 hours	10–18 hours	18–28 hours
Lente	1–3 hours	10–18 hours	24–36 hours
Protamine Zinc	3–7 hours	15–22 hours	24–36 hours
Ultralente	5–8 hours	16–24 hours	28–36 hours

cardiac pain or can be referred to epigastrium, back, arms, and upper thorax.

b. **Etiology**
    - Age-related degenerative changes
    - Weakened tissue wall between esophagus and diaphragm
    - Increased abdominal pressure (strain from forceful vomiting)
    - Obesity

c. **Clinical Manifestations**
    - Burning pain or pressure at xiphoid process worsened by coughing, sneezing, bending, and reclining
    - Severe tightening pain
    - Heartburn, sour stomach
    - Dysphagia, belching, regurgitation
    - Possible bleeding

d. **Multidisciplinary Approaches**
    - Dietary modification (low calorie, low residue)
    - Weight reduction if indicated
    - Antacid therapy (see Table 5.6); antacids neutralize gastric acidity and relieve indigestion and similar GI symptoms. The high inci-

Table 5.6 Antacids

Examples	Common Side Effects	Nursing Implications
Aluminum hydroxide	Constipation, nausea, vomiting	Monitor serum electrolytes. Advise patient to take with large amounts of fluids.
Calcium carbonate	Constipation, nausea Rebound hyperactivity Milk-alkali syndrome	Warn patient against taking with milk or foods high in vitamin D.
Sodium bicarbonate	Fluid retention, belching, alkalosis, hypercalcemia, hyperphosphatemia, nausea, vomiting, headache, confusion	Caution patients on a sodium-restricted diet about antacid use. Highest sodium content: Delcid, Di-Gel, Simeco, Titralac, Trisogel. Warn against taking with milk or foods high in vitamin D.
Magnesium carbonate	Severe diarrhea	Monitor intake and output. Correct diarrhea promptly.

Interactions: all antacids
Decrease the effects of barbiturates, chlorpromazine, digoxin, iron preparations, isoniazid, nitrofurantoin, oral anticoagulants, para-aminosalicyclic acid, penicillins, phenytoin, phenylbutazone, salicylates, sulfonamides, tetracyclines, vitamins A and C.

Aluminum hydroxide increases effects of meperidine, pseudoephedrine.

dence of GI symptoms among the elderly make antacids a widely used, self-prescribed group of drugs.

Additional Nursing Care That Can Be Incorporated into the Generic Care Plan

- Educate patient to appropriate diet, assist in keeping a food diary and identifying eating patterns and preferences.
- Withhold food for at least 2 hours prior to bedtime or a nap; symptoms increase in recumbent position so elevate head of bed slightly during sleep.
- Observe for and prevent aspiration; be aware that a report of night cough can indicate that aspiration is occurring during sleep.
- Evaluate success of antacid therapy and observe for side effects (e.g., diarrhea, constipation, hypercalcemia, hypernatremia).
- Be alert to the possibility of myocardial infarction if symptoms do not subside with treatment of antacids (changes in blood pressure and ECG that do not occur with hiatal hernia; angina is more closely associated with activity).

GENERIC CARE PLAN FOR THE NURSING DIAGNOSIS
FLUID VOLUME EXCESS

1. General Information

Fluid volume excess is a state of vascular, cellular, or extracellular fluid overload. Additional fluids place an added burden on older hearts, which tend to be less efficient at managing such stresses. Peripheral edema is more of a problem for the elderly due to the diminished peripheral perfusion often present; this can threaten skin integrity and result in ulcer formation. Fluid volume excess most often is manifested by edema, an accumulation of fluid in cells, tissues, or body cavities. When edema is bilateral, cardiac problems are most likely responsible.

a. Etiology
- Decreased cardiac output (e.g., associated with congestive heart failure, myocardial infarction)
- Liver disease
- Renal failure
- Steroid therapy
- Hormonal disturbances (e.g., pituitary, adrenal)
- Excess fluid intake (e.g., IV therapy)
- Excess sodium intake
- Dependent venous pooling or venostasis
- Inadequate lymphatic drainage
- See Table 5.7 for common fluid and electrolyte imbalances

b. Clinical Manifestations
- Evidence of swelling (increased circumference of extremities; puffiness of fingers, feet, and around eyes; ability to indent edematous area)
- Weakness, fatigue
- Rhonchi, rales, cough
- Weight increase

Table 5.7 Common Fluid and Electrolyte Imbalances

Imbalance	Cause	Signs and Symptoms
Dehydration	Fluid loss from vomiting, diarrhea, polyuria, excessive perspiration or drainage	Anorexia, nausea, vomiting, apathy, weakness, weight loss, postural hypotension, sunken eyes, poor skin turgor, temperature elevation, weak/rapid pulse, decreased urine output, increased specific gravity of urine, increased hematocrit
Overhydration	Congestive heart failure, cirrhosis, nephrosis, rapid infusion of IV fluids	Edema, ascites, effusion, dyspnea, elevated pulse, pulmonary congestion
Hyponatremia (sodium level below 135 mEq/liter)	Excessive fluid intake, vomiting, gastric suctioning	Confusion, lethargy, anorexia, nausea, vomiting, seizures, coma
Hypernatremia (sodium level above 145 mEq/liter)	Excessive fluid loss or inadequate fluid intake	Thirst, confusion, weakness, irritability, poor skin turgor, increased temperature, decreased urine output, increased specific gravity of urine, decreased blood pressure
Hypokalemia (potassium level below 3.4 mEq/liter)	Diarrhea, vomiting, NG suctioning, urinary loss, insufficient potassium intake	Weakness, irritability, anorexia, nausea, decreased reflexes, dysrhythmias
Hyperkalemia (potassium level above 5 mEq/liter)	Acute renal failure, GI bleeding, increased tissue injury or breakdown, acidosis	Weaknesses, paresthesias, paralysis, decreased pulse and blood pressure, cardiac arrest
Metabolic Acidosis (bicarbonate level below 20 mEq/liter)	Diabetic ketoacidosis, starvation, puremia, salicylate toxicity	Hyperventilation, lowered pCO_2
Metabolic Alkalosis (bicarbonate level above 33 mEq/liter)	Vomiting, NG suctioning, diuretic therapy	Depressed respirations, tetany

- Taut, shiny skin, possibly cracked, weepy
- Increased blood pressure or pulse volume in affected extremity
- Fluid intake exceeds output
- Jugular venous distension

c. **Multidisciplinary Approaches**
   - Diagnose and treat underlying cause
   - Dietary modification: sodium restriction
   - Medications: diuretics, potassium supplements

2. Nursing Process

a. **Assessment**
   - Vital signs, daily weight, I&O
   - Circumference of extremities and abdominal girth
   - Amount of pitting at various sites

b. **Goals**
   Patient
   - will reduce the amount of edema and be protected from complications.
   - will regain/maintain fluid balance.

c. **Interventions**
   - Carefully monitor IV infusions particularly if patient is confused; ensure IV rate is not subject to positional changes.
   - Change positions frequently and elevate edematous extremity.
   - Use low semi-Fowler's position to minimize pressure on diaphragm.
   - Restrict sodium intake, offer salt substitutes, if appropriate.
   - Provide good skin care.
   - If on diuretics, monitor output carefully, ensure bathroom facilities are close and safely available.
   - Avoid rapid mobilization of severe edema (profound intoxication can occur from the metabolic debris carried in the fluids).
   - Monitor administration of diuretics carefully for desired results, possible side effects.

d. **Evaluation**
   - Patient's
     • fluid and electrolyte balance is maintained/restored.
     • abdominal girth and circumference of extremities return to normal.
     • weight gained by fluid retention is lost.
     • skin remains intact.

e. **Possible Related Nursing Diagnoses**
Alteration in tissue perfusion (peripheral)
Impaired physical mobility
Impairment of skin integrity
Potential for infection

GENERIC CARE PLAN FOR THE NURSING DIAGNOSIS
FLUID VOLUME DEFICIT

1. General Information

Dehydration is a condition in which there is a reduction in body fluids. It poses a significant threat for the elderly because a decrease in body fluids occurs as a result of aging; thus, their reserves are less. The decreased thirst sensation present in the elderly also increases their risk of this problem.

a. **Etiology**
    – Excess fluid loss (e.g., polyuria, abnormal drainage, diarrhea, vomiting)
    – Increased metabolic rate (e.g., fever)
    – Lack of adequate fluid intake (confused, depressed, unconscious, unable to reach or drink fluids)
    – Medications (diuretics, laxatives, sedatives)
    – See Table 5.7 for common fluid and electrolyte imbalances

b. **Clinical Manifestations**
    – Change in mental status
    – Dryness of lips, oral mucosa, conjunctiva
    – Poor skin turgor
    – Shrunken, furrowed tongue (usually develops in late stage)
    – Increased temperature
    – Decreased blood pressure
    – Decreased urine output

c. **Multidisciplinary Approaches**
    – Parenteral administration of fluids and electrolytes and/or tube feedings

2. Nursing Process

a. **Assessment**
    – Vital signs, weight
    – Fluid intake and output

b. **Etiology**
- Prolonged pressure against bony prominence leading to tissue anoxia and ischemia
- Shearing force
  - sitting up in bed
  - being pulled across bed
- Vitamin C deficiency
- Anemia, hypoproteinemia

c. **Three Stages of Development**
- *Hyperemia*: Localized redness, leaves when pressure is removed and tissue circulation restored.
- *Ischemia*: Discoloration and swelling of skin; occurs after 6 or more hours of continuous pressure or sooner in a debilitated patient.
- *Ulceration*: Open lesion exposing subcutaneous tissue.
- *Necrosis*: Dead skin that may extend through fascia and bone; eschar is often present.

d. **Multidisciplinary Approaches**
- Debridement done mechanically, surgically, or chemically
- Proteolytic enzymes such as Elase or Travase ointments
- Treatments to promote granulation and epitheliazation including oxygen under pressure, dry heat, gelfoam powder, gold leaf or sugar, electrical stimulation, whirlpool

Additional Nursing Care That Can Be Incorporated into the Generic Care Plan

- All stages
  - Determine cause, stage, and type of ulcer
  - Position patient off affected area
  - Keep dressings clean and intact
  - Assure adequate nutritional intake
  - Monitor healing progress
  - Observe for signs of infection and related complications.
- Stage 1: hyperemia
  - Cover reddened area with protective dressing, such as Op-site or Duoderm, and adhesive foam.
- Stage 2: ischemia
  - Cover reddened area with protective dressing of Vigilon, applied jelly side down.
  - Cover with adhesive foam cut to fit in the area.
  - Clean wound daily with saline or solution of choice.
- Stage 3: ulceration
  - Cover ulcer with transparent dressing that is permeable to oxygen and water vapor.
  - Cover with adhesive foam doughnut.

- Allow exudate to accumulate under dressing (this provides moisture necessary for epidermal regeneration); aspirate drainage only if it threatens to break dressing seal.
  - Stage 4: necrosis
    - Remove eschar. Chemical debridement (using products such as Elase or Travase) is slower, but reduces the risks of sepsis and bleeding associated with surgical debridement; chemical debriders should be discontinued as soon as eschar disappears.
    - Follow prescribed treatment plan to facilitate healing, which could include
      * topical applications: drainage absorbers, monosaccharides, heavy metal ions
      * oxygenation: by direct appliction to the ulcer using a face mask, or within a hyperboric chamber
      * ultrasound: directed at ulcer to break down cellular obstructions and increase local circulation
    - Evaluate the need for special beds that are available under Medicare under certain conditions (e.g., Clinetron, Mediscus, Mark IV).

GENERIC CARE PLAN FOR THE NURSING DIAGNOSIS
ALTERATION IN ORAL MUCOUS MEMBRANE

1. General Information

Alteration in oral mucous membrane is a potential or actual interruption in the integrity of the layers and/or protective properties of the oral mucosa. Health status of the oral cavity has a significant impact on dietary intake, self-image, speech and communication, socialization, and general health.

a. Etiology
- Reduced saliva production
- Atrophy of the mucosal epithelium, increasing risk of irritation and infection
- Ill-fitting dentures
- Years of smoking, drinking
- Limited ability to floss, brush, or clean dentures because of decreased manual dexterity
- Poor dentition

b. Clinical Manifestations
- Lips: fissures, lesions, ulcers, discoloration, dryness, assymetry
- Tongue: ulcers, unusually raised papillae, fissures, smoothness, pain, coating, white patchy areas, limited motion

- Gums and mucous membrane: ulcers, fissures, white patchy areas, masses, swelling, numbness, bleeding, friction rubs from teeth or dentures
- Teeth: decay, brittleness, looseness, jagged edges
- Decreased appetite and weight loss

c. **Multidisciplinary Approaches**
  - Correction of dental problems
    • remove loose, broken, diseased teeth
    • repair dentures
  - Differential diagnosis to identify infections, cancerous lesions

2. Nursing Process

a. **Assessment**
  - Integrity of oral cavity
  - Fit, condition, and cleanliness of dentures
  - Pattern of oral hygiene, last dental visit
  - Halitosis, change in eating patterns, types of food

b. **Goal**
  Patient will reestablish/maintain good oral hygiene and healthy gums, teeth, lips and tongue.

c. **Interventions**
  - When natural teeth are present
    • brush at least twice daily (preferably after each meal) with a soft nylon brush.
    • use short strokes, holding the brush at a 45° angle with the gums, and moving from the gum to the crown of the tooth.
    • brush the tongue and roof of the mouth gently.
    • if arthritis or other conditions interfere with normal manipulation of a toothbrush, explore the use of electric or battery-operated toothbrushes, or adapt the brush by padding the handle (an occupational therapist can be a valuable resource for matching adaptive equipment to the individual patient).
    • floss at least twice daily, gently bringing floss between gum and tooth; floss holders are available to ease flossing in difficult-to-reach areas or when only one hand is functional.
    • be aware that Water Piks and similar water jet sprays are not recommended for older adults because they can spray bacteria onto unhealthy gums, leading to serious infection; however, if patient has healthy gums, use of a Pik should not be discouraged.
  - When dentures are present
    • remove and insert dentures over basin of water to prevent breakage if they should fall accidentally.

- grasp palate and front surface of dentures on both sides and gently pull from gum until seal is broken and denture is easily removed.
- place dentures in denture cup or plastic container and cover with a nonabrasive cleaning agent (commercial preparations are available to clean dentures and remove stains) but homemade mixtures can be equally effective and less expensive: 1 tablespoon bleach and 1 tablespoon Calgon in 8 ounces of water; or 1 teaspoon ammonia in 8 ounces of water; or 1 teaspoon vinegar in 8 ounces of water).
- soak dentures in solution for 15 minutes then scrub with a toothbrush to remove particles.
- have patient rinse mouth and brush gums with a soft toothbrush while dentures are out.
- remove denture adhesive thoroughly from dentures and gums to avoid irritation and infection.
- remove dentures at night to prevent chronic pressure on the soft tissue; whenever dentures are out of the mouth soak them in water, homemade solution; or a commercial preparation to prevent warping.
- suggest that the patient's name or social security number be engraved on the dentures as a means of identification.

d. Evaluation
    – Client's oral mucosa is moist, a healthy pink color, and free from breaks and irritation.

e. Possible Related Nursing Diagnoses
Alteration in comfort
Alteration in nutrition
Knowledge deficit regarding oral hygiene
Potential for infection

References

Beattie, B., & Louie, V. (1983). Nutrition and health in the elderly. In W. Reichel (Ed.), *Clinical aspects of aging* (2nd ed.). Baltimore: Williams & Wilkins.

Bennett, P. (1984). Diabetes in the elderly: Diagnosis and epidemiology. *Geriatrics, 38*(5), 36–44.

Bloomer, J. (1983). Managing cirrhosis in the geriatric patient. *Geriatrics, 38*(11), 66–74.

Cassell, B. (1986). Treating pressure sores stage by stage. *RN, 49*(1), 36–40.

Cooney, T., & Reuler, J. (1983). Protecting the elderly from pressure sores. *Geriatrics, 38*(2), 125–134.

Eliopoulos, C. (1984). Assessment of the gastrointestinal system. In C. Eliopoulos (Ed.), *Health assessment of the older adult.* Menlo Park, CA: Addison-Wesley.

Helfand, A. (1983). Foot health for the elderly. In W. Reichel (Ed.), *Clinical aspects of aging* (2nd ed.). Baltimore: Williams & Wilkins.

Hudis, M. (1983). Dentistry for the elderly. In W. Reichel (Ed.), *Clinical aspects of aging* (2nd ed.). Baltimore: Williams & Wilkins.

Joachem, G. (1983). How to give a great foot massage. *Geriatric Nursing, 4*(1), 28–29.

Korting, G. (1980). *Geriatric dermatology.* Philadelphia: Saunders.

Kravitz, S. (1983). Anemia in the elderly. In W. Reichel (Ed.), *Clinical aspects of aging* (2nd ed.). Baltimore: Williams & Wilkins.

Lindeman, R. (1983). Application of fluid and electrolyte balance principles to the older patient. In W. Reichel (Ed.), *Clinical aspects of aging* (2nd ed.). Baltimore: Williams & Wilkins.

Mangieri, D. (1982). Saving your elderly patient's skin. *Nursing 82, 12*(10), 44–45.

Masoro, E. (1985). Nutrition and aging—A current assessment. *Journal of Nutrition, 115*(7), 842–8.

Nelder, K. (1984). Nutrition, aging and the skin. *Geriatrics, 39*(2), 69–88.

Overton, M., & Lukert, B. (1977). *Clinical nutrition. A physiologic approach.* Chicago: Year Book Medical Publishers.

Palmer, R. (1984). Fluid and electrolyte disorders. In C. Cassel & J. Walsh (Eds.), *Geriatric medicine, Vol I.* New York: Springer.

Price, J. (1979). Oral health care for the geriatric patient. *Journal of Gerontological Nursing, 5*(2), 25–29.

Reddy, M. (1983). Decubitus ulcers: Principles of prevention and management. *Geriatrics, 38*(7), 55–64.

Roe, D. (1983). *Geriatric nutrition.* Englewood Cliffs, NJ: Prentice Hall.

Smith, F. (1984). Gastroenterology. In C. Cassel & J. Walsh (Eds.), *Geriatric medicine, Vol I.* New York: Springer.

Stuckey, W. (1983). Common anemias: A practical guide to diagnosis and management. *Geriatrics, 38*(8), 42–47.

Zerber, N., Miller, S., & Demuth, R. (1982). Decubitus ulcers. *Asepses, 4*(5), 19–23.

CHAPTER 6

ELIMINATION
FUNCTIONAL HEALTH PATTERN

Elimination problems, common among the elderly, provoke anxiety and distress for both the individual and the nurse. Many factors contribute to these problems in old age. The tendency to consume less bulk and fluids and reduced activity levels heighten the risk of constipation imposed by slower peristalsis. Diminished nerve sensation to the lower bowel can reduce the signal of the need to defecate. Reduced bladder capacity can increase the frequency of urination, and weaker muscles along the urinary tract can cause urinary retention, dribbling, and stress incontinence to become greater risks. Enlarged prostate glands, urinary tract infections, calculi, altered mental status, and other problems more prevalent in the older population can promote incontinence. Medications can impact bowel and bladder elimination in a variety of ways. Toileting habits, environmental factors, and functional capacity also contribute to elimination problems. There is a loss of dignity and self-esteem when aged persons have difficulty controlling their bodily functions, not to mention the risks to comfort, skin integrity, and general well-being. An essential nursing role is to facilitate the reestablishment and maintenance of normal elimination patterns.

GENERIC CARE PLAN FOR THE NURSING DIAGNOSIS
ALTERATION IN BOWEL ELIMINATION: CONSTIPATION

1. General Information

Constipation is the abnormal delay or infrequent passage of dry, hardened feces. It is one of the greatest problems for the elderly. The colon can lose innervation and experience smooth muscle atrophy. Laxatives need to be chosen carefully, considering the specific action of the medication and the cause of the constipation.

a. **Etiology**
    – Inactivity and/or decrease in activity
    – Poor bowel habits
        • not establishing regular pattern or time
        • ignoring signal for elimination
    – Poor nutrition
        • an inadequate intake of bulk related to limited ability to purchase and prepare proper foods
        • self-imposed fluid restrictions related to concern about urinary frequency
    – Emotional problems
        • depression can reduce food intake, promote inactivity
        • boredom, withdrawal, isolation
        • anorexia, which may be physical or emotional in origin
    – Drugs
        • iron preparations
        • antihypertensives
        • analgesics
        • tranquilizers
        • anticholinergics
        • antacids containing calcium carbonate
        • laxatives (excessive use can cause muscular atony, decreased awareness of the presence of stool)
    – Organic problems
        • hypothyroidism, hypercalcemia
        • tumors
        • diabetic neuropathy
        • hypokalemia
        • anorectal lesions, hemorrhoids
        • ischemia of the colon
        • decreased motility of the GI tract
        • dementia
        • hemorrhoids, fissures
        • colon stricture, voluulus

b. **Clinical Manifestations**
    – Difficult passage of hard, dry stool
    – Decreased frequency of bowel movements
    – Abdominal fullness, discomfort, flatulence/distention
    – Hard stool in rectum on palpation
    – Nausea, vomiting, anorexia

c. **Multidisciplinary Approaches**
    – Dietary adjustments, exercise
    – Laxatives, stool softener (see Table 6.1)

Table 6.1   Laxatives

Categories	Examples	Action	Nursing Implications
Bulk former	Methylcellulose Psyllium	Absorb water in intestines and expand, creating more bulk. This extra bulk distends the intestines and increases peristalsis.	Good fluid intake necessary to prevent intestinal obstruction. Effects *usually* noted in 12–24 hours. Do not use when intestinal obstruction, abdominal pain, dehydration, nausea, or vomiting are suspected or present. Not absorbed systemically.
Stool softeners	Docusate calcium Docusate sodium	Promote collection of fluid in stool, creating a softer stool mass and eases bowel movements	Carefully evaluate use with patients who have cardiac, renal, or other problems impairing management of excess fluid. Effects usually noted in 24–48 hours. Do not stimulate peristalsis: more effective as prevention rather than cure. Absorbed systemically.
Hyper-osmolar	Glycerin Magnesium salts Saline	Pull fluid into the colon (salt-based laxatives also draw fluid to the small intestine) causing bowel distension, increased peristalsis.	Glycerin is administered as a suppository or enema; can cause cramps. Ensure good fluid intake with administration of magnesium salts. Effects usually noted within 1–3 hours. Avoid magnesium salts in patients with abdominal pain, serious cardiac problems, renal disease, intestinal obstruction, nausea, vomiting, or fecal impaction. Do not administer *any* medication 2 hours before or after saline laxative because saline interferes with absorption. Magnesium salts are absorbed systematically; if used on a long-term basis, periodically evaluate serum electrolytes.
Stimulants	Cascara Sagrada Senna	Irritate smooth muscle of intestine to increase peristalsis; draw fluid into small intestine and colon to distend bowel, further increasing peristalsis.	Use on short-term basis only; long-term use can cause electrolyte imbalance, particularly hypokalemia. Effects are usually noted within 6–10 hours (senna is more potent than cascara). Cascara can discolor urine (advise patient). Avoid use in patients with nausea, vomiting, intestinal obstruction, abdominal pain, or fecal impaction. Some systemic absorption.
Lubricants	Mineral oil	Coats fecal matter and prevents	Avoid use in patients with nausea, vomiting, intestinal

(continued)

Table 6.1   Laxatives (continued)

Categories	Examples	Action	Nursing Implications
		absorption of fluid from feces, resulting in easier passage of stool.	obstruction, abdominal pain, or fecal impaction. Administer on an empty stomach as it will delay emptying. Effects usually noted within 6–8 hours. Minimize unpleasant taste by having patient hold ice chips on tongue prior to administration or by mixing with soda or juice. Not recommended for older persons due to serious complications that can result in –dehydration from diarrhea –lipid pneumonias and lung abscesses from aspiration –deficiencies of fat-soluble vitamins A, D, K, and E (dissolved in and excreted with the oil). Emulsified oil is absorbed more completely than nonemulsified.

- Readjust medications
- Treat depression and organic disease
- Enemas

2. Nursing Process

a. Assessment
- Client's definition of constipation (many adults, due to cultural norms, sometimes interpret the lack of a daily bowel movement as constipation despite absence of clinical signs)
- Dietary, medicinal, activity, and elimination habits
  - have patient keep a diary of food/fluid intake, bowel movements and activity
  - ask about the use of laxatives, suppositories, enemas, and other methods used to facilitate elimination
  - take a thorough drug history, including use of over-the-counter medications
- Recent losses, changes, or events that could have impacted on physical or emotional status, e.g., retirement, need for prolonged bedrest, death of loved one, new medical disorder, other drastic changes or losses, presence of depression
- Palpate abdomen; auscultate bowel sounds
- Character and frequency of stools

– Presence of other symptoms that, when associated with constipation, could indicate larger problems
  • alternating constipation and diarrhea (tumors, irritable colon,
    fecal impaction)
  • nausea and vomiting (diverticulitis, bowel obstruction)
  • low back pain (irritable colon), rectal pain, fissures
  • thin stools (diverticular disease, irritable colon, hemorrhoids,
    rectal cancer)
  • intolerance to cold, weight gain, hoarseness, slowed mental func-
    tion (hypothyroidism)
  • bloody stools (hemorrhoids, ulcerative colitis, diverticulitis, im-
    paction, colon cancer)

b. Goal
Patient will
– reestablish good bowel function without excessive dependence on
  laxatives.
– learn ways to prevent constipation and appropriate interventions
  to alleviate constipation.

c. Interventions
– Encourage change in dietary habits such as
  • increase dietary fiber and bulk (bran, whole grains, raw vege-
    tables)
  • introduce foods that may induce elimination (prunes, chocolate,
    spinach)
  • ask patient about foods that have produced loose stools in the
    past and incorporate them in diet in moderation
  • increase fluid intake if not contraindicated (e.g., CHF)
– Increase general activity level and encourage regular exercise on
  a daily basis.
– Teach patient to develop good bowel habits such as
  • attending to physiologic cues
  • toileting regularly at times when success is most likely after break-
    fast; the introduction of food following night-time inactivity stim-
    ulates the GI tract
– Wean from laxatives or enemas if indicated and if muscle tone is
  adequate.
– Be aware that patient may be unable to empty bowel at one sitting
  • have patient try a second bowel movement, 30-45 minutes after
    the first
  • alert staff to take requests for second toiletings seriously
  • use digital stimulation
– Provide privacy and time alone to defecate
– Avoid using a bedpan if at all possible with a bedridden patient,
  because it forces the extension of legs, abdominal hyperextension,
  defecation without muscular help, and causes undue strain; if the

patient is not properly positioned, gravity may impede passage of stool
- Use a commode chair or toilet when patient is able, to promote relaxation
- Teach techniques to facilitate elimination
  - elevate feet slightly (using small foot rest or book)
  - lean forward (increases abdominal pressure)
- Remember that straining or enemas can stimulate the vagus nerve thus inhibiting heart function (Valsalva maneuver)

d. Evaluation
- Patient
  - regularly passes formed stool with no or minimal difficulty or pain.
  - has bowel movements without inducement by laxatives, suppositories, or enemas.

e. Possible Related Nursing Diagnoses
Alteration in nutrition: less than body requirements
Impaired physical mobility
Self-care deficit: toileting

Selected Health Problems Frequently Associated with the Nursing Diagnosis ALTERATION IN BOWEL ELIMINATION: CONSTIPATION

1. Fecal Impaction

a. Definition
A large accumulation of feces in the rectum or colon that is difficult to move. It is the most common reason for nonacute intestinal obstruction. Colorectal cancer and cardiac disease are relative contraindications to manually removing an impaction.

b. Etiology
- Stress
- Lack of privacy
- Irregular evacuation patterns
- Dehydration
- Decreased motility of GI tract
- Organic disease or impaired mental functions
- Painful defecation (anal fissures/hemorrhoids)
- Sensory/motor disorders (CVA, neurologic diseases)
- Side effects of drugs (antacids, iron, barium, aluminum, calcium)

c. **Clinical Manifestations**
   - Absence of regular bowel movement
   - Abdominal fullness and discomfort
   - Oozing of fecal material from rectum (sometimes resembling diarrhea)
   - Poor appetite
   - Lethargy
   - Fecal mass on digital exam

d. **Multidisciplinary Approaches**
   - Manual removal of impaction
   - Laxatives, enemas (see Table 6.1)

Additional Nursing Care That Can Be Incorporated into the Generic Care Plan

   - Prepare patient for removal of fecal impaction
     • explain procedure
     • postion patient on left side with knees flexed; drape appropriately
     • ask patient to take deep breaths to diminish effects of Valsalva maneuver.
   - Remove impaction
     • insert lubricated, gloved finger into rectum using a circular motion; remove small masses
     • if mass is large, insert 2 lubricated, gloved fingers and break up mass before removing
     • talk with patient throughout procedure; encourage relaxation.
   - Utilize other measures, as necessary
     • oil retention enemas (if not contraindicated)
     • hydrogen peroxide (50-100 cc through a rectal tube).
   - Record the results, patient tolerance, any problems noted.
   - Institute measures to prevent recurrence; monitor bowel habits.

2. Hemorrhoids

a. **Definition**
   A mass of dilated veins in swollen tissue situated near the anal sphincter. They can develop in old age or be a problem from earlier years.

b. **Etiology**
   - Chronic constipation
   - Heavy lifting
   - Straining when defecating
   - Long periods of standing or sitting
   - Obesity
   - Portal hypertension

c. **Clinical Manifestations**
   - Perineal itching
   - Bleeding during or after bowel movements
   - Pain
   - Bulge in rectal area
   - Swollen, dilated perianal veins

d. **Multidisciplinary Approaches**
   - Dietary modification (low residue, high fiber to keep feces soft)
   - Topical anesthetics and hemorrhoid preparations
   - Stool softeners (see Table 6.1)
   - Sitz baths
   - Surgical intervention (hemorroidectomy)

Additional Nursing Care That Can Be Incorporated into the Generic Care Plan

- Relieve discomfort and pain with warm sitz baths
  • measure water temperature carefully since the elderly are more susceptible to burns
  • observe for dizziness caused by lowered blood pressure (blood tends to be pulled to lower extremity during sitz bath).
  • provide assistance to prevent falls
- Teach proper diet to prevent constipation.
- Teach avoidance of straining and sitting on toilet for long periods, and care of anal area with compresses and ointments.

3. Diverticulosis

a. **Definition**
   A condition in which there are multiple pouches along the intestinal wall. Diverticulitis is the inflammation of the diverticula. They usually develop in the fifth decade of life and increase in size and number as the years advance if left untreated.

b. **Etiology**
   - Obesity
   - Low-residue diet
   - Chronic constipation
   - Hiatal hernia
   - Genetic disposition

c. **Clinical Manifestations**
   - Lower left quadrant pain and cramps
   - Flatulence
   - Nausea and vomiting

– Fever
– Bowel irregularity

d. **Multidisciplinary Approaches**
– High-fiber, low-residue diet
– Bulk laxatives, stool softeners, mineral oil (see Table 6.1)
– Antibiotics (see Table 4.1)
– Surgical intervention (colon resection)

Additional Nursing Care That Can Be Incorporated into the Generic Care Plan

– Relieve pain (see Chapter 8, Pain).
– Teach diet modification.
– Prevent diverticulitis (see Chapter 4, Infection).
– Teach how to avoid intra-abdominal pressure by avoiding straining at stool, vomiting, lifting and restrictive clothing.

4. Colon Cancer

a. **Definition**
A malignant neoplasm originating in the large intestine. It is the second most common cause of death in the United States. A majority of cases of colon cancer occur in people 50 years of age or older; it affects both sexes equally. Most cancers of the large intestine (75%) occur in the descending colon, rectosigmoid, or rectum. Cancer occurring in the ascending colon has different clinical manifestations from that occurring in the descending colon.

b. **Etiology**
– Unknown; incidence increases with age
– Familial polyposis; chronic ulcerative colitis
– Higher incidence where diet is low in fiber and high in refined carbohydrates

c. **Clinical Manifestations**
– Left-sided mass
  • weight loss
  • narrow, ribbonlike stools
  • rectal bleeding
  • rectal mass
  • mucus discharge
  • changes in bowel habit
– Right-sided mass
  • usually asymptomatic
  • weakness and fatigue
  • occult bleeding

- diarrhea
- palpable mass
- anemia
- complaints of vague abdominal pain

d. Multidisciplinary Approaches
  - Radiation and chemotherapy (palliative treatment to shrink the tumor)
  - Surgery
    - Ascending colon: right colectomy with ileotransverse anatomosis
    - Descending colon: left colectomy with reanastomosis of transverse colon
    - Distal sigmoid and rectum: abdominal-perineal/resection with permanent colostomy

Additional Nursing Care That Can Be Incorporated into the Generic Care Plan

  - Discuss planned surgery with patient; include content re colostomy, appearance and location of stoma.
  - Evaluate physical ability to do ostomy care (e.g., ability to use hands, fingers; eyesight; physical strength; willingness to learn).
  - Encourage patient to express fears, grief, and anxiety concerning diagnosis and treatment.
  - Allow patient to regain physical and emotional strength before beginning postoperative teaching regarding ostomy care, diet.
  - Teach patient complications to observe for and report
    - pain, redness, swelling
    - excoriated peristomal skin of incision
    - obstruction of output
    - stoma prolapse or retraction
    - altered stool consistency
  - Provide patient with written instructions concerning
    - dietary considerations about foods that cause flatus (cabbage, beans, carbonated beverages) and blockage (nuts, spinach, lettuce, popcorn)
    - ostomy appliances: how to measure for size, where to buy
    - community resources (ostomy clubs)
  - Give ostomy care as indicated.

GENERIC CARE PLAN FOR THE NURSING DIAGNOSIS
ALTERATION IN BOWEL ELIMINATION: DIARRHEA

1. General Information

Diarrhea is an increase in the amount and frequency of bowel movements. When diarrhea results from an infection, stools are watery and loose.

Sometimes the rapid expulsion of stools causes a lack of bowel control or fecal incontinence, which improves when the diarrhea ceases.

a. **Etiology**
   – Bacterial, viral, or parasitic infection
   – Drug reaction (e.g., antibiotics, laxatives)
   – Enzyme deficiency
   – Food allergy
   – Stress
   – Diverticulosis
   – Cancer
   – Nutritional supplements and enteral feedings
   – Malabsorption, vitamin deficiency

b. **Clinical Manifestations**
   – Increased frequency and volume of stool
   – Watery stool
   – Abdominal cramping
   – Nausea and vomiting
   – Malaise, possible fever
   – Dehydration
   – Positive stool, blood culture
   – Altered mental status, confusion

c. **Multidisciplinary Approaches**
   – Treatment of underlying cause
   – Replacement of fluids and electrolytes
   – Antidiarrheals or fewer laxatives

2. Nursing Process

a. **Assessment**
   – Clinical manifestations including onset and frequency
   – Possible causative factors (e.g., travel history, drug regimens)
   – Symptoms of electrolyte imbalance (see Table 5.7)

b. **Goals**
   Patient
   – will reestablish normal bowel movements if possible.
   – will decrease frequency of bowel movements.
   – will remain free from dehydration, weakness, or anal excoriation.

c. **Interventions**
   – Record I&O, number and character of stools, daily weight.
   – Consider diarrhea as a sign of infection until cause is determined; follow enteric precautions and monitor vital signs.
   – Practice proper hand washing before and after contact with pa-

tient; cleanse rectal area, apply petroleum gel to prevent excoriation.
  – Observe for signs of dehydration (e.g., poor skin turgor, postural hypotension, sunken eyes, rapid pulse); increase intake of fluids as tolerated, avoiding milk products.
  – Admininster IV fluids, electrolytes, as ordered.
  – Administer antidiarrheal agents as ordered; observe for change in stools, color, amount, consistency.
  – Teach patient practices to avoid or control diarrhea (e.g., dietary practices, safe laxative use).

d. Evaluation
  – Patient
    • establishes normal elimination pattern
    • maintains normal perirectal skin integrity.
    • has normal skin turgor and serum electrolyte values.
    • is free from postural hypotension.

e. Possible Related Nursing Diagnoses
Fluid volume deficit
Impaired skin integrity

GENERIC CARE PLAN FOR THE NURSING DIAGNOSIS
ALTERATION IN BOWEL ELIMINATION: INCONTINENCE

1. General Information

Fecal incontinence refers to the inability to control bowel movements due to physical or cognitive impairment. Chronic incontinence of feces, which can appear as diarrhea, is usually associated with a neurologic deficit or disease of the colon, rectum, or anus.

a. Etiology
  – Constipation, fecal impaction
  – Carcinoma of the rectum
  – Prolapsed rectum
  – Debilitation and weakness causing the inability to exert muscular effort against a normal gastrocolic reflex
  – Severe diarrhea
  – Inability to toilet independently
  – Cognitive deficit

b. Clinical Manifestations
  – Uncontrolled passage of fecal matter
  – Neurogenic incontinence (causes incontinence once or twice a day)

c. **Multidisciplinary Approaches**
   - Identification and treatment of underlying cause
   - Bowel retraining program (see Table 6.2)

2. Nursing Process

a. **Assessment**
   - Frequency, characteristics, precipitating factors, and amount of stool associated with each episode of incontinence
   - Awareness of sensations signaling the need to defecate
   - Presence of impaction, masses

b. **Goals**
   Patient
   - will regain bowel control and maintain regular elimination pattern.
   - will be free from skin breakdown.

Table 6.2 Bowel Retraining

Purpose
   To reestablish partial to full control of bowel movements.

Assessment
   Client's general physical and mental condition
   Bowel and sphincter function
   Cause, length of time, and degree of incontinence
   Anticipated cooperation of patient and family

Preliminary Actions
   Keep record of patient's bowel movement pattern: time, amount of stool, relationship to meals and activities.
   Identify stimuli for bowel movement.
   Identify patient's ability to perceive the need to have bowel movement.

Procedure
   Based upon assessments, establish regular time when bowel movement can be anticipated and plan toileting at that time.
   Insert a glycerin suppository into rectum approximately 30 minutes prior to scheduled time.
   Position patient in sitting position on bedpan or commode, out of bed if possible.
   Place footstool under feet to promote bowel elimination.
   Instruct patient to take several deep breaths, tighten abdomen, press hands on abdomen to apply pressure and bear down, bending down also helps if patient can tolerate it.
   If there is no bowel movement after 10 minutes take patient off bedpan or commode.
   Maintain a record of attempts and outcomes.
   After a routine is established, mechanical stimulation through the use of a suppository may not be necessary.

c. **Interventions**
   - Record frequency, amount, and patient's control of bowel movements.
   - Assure proper hygienic practices and thorough skin cleaning after bowel movements; keep skin clean and dry.
   - Establish bowel retraining program (see Table 6.2) if appropriate for patient.

d. **Evaluation**
   - Patient
     • establishes control of bowel movements, if possible.
     • Maintains normal skin integrity around rectal area, buttocks.

e. **Possible Related Nursing Diagnoses**
   Anxiety
   Disturbance in self-concept
   Impaired skin integrity
   Potential for infection
   Self-care deficit: toileting
   Social isolation

GENERIC CARE PLAN FOR THE NURSING DIAGNOSIS
ALTERATION IN PATTERNS OF URINARY ELIMINATION: INCONTINENCE

1. General Information

Urinary incontinence is the inability to control the passage of urine. Although not a normal outcome of aging, incontinence is more prevalent among older persons.

   - Stress incontinence occurs due to a weakness of supporting pelvic muscles that causes urine to be released through the bladder outlet when one coughs, laughs, sneezes, or during exercise.
   - Urge incontinence is due to a sudden urge produced by spasm or irritated bladder walls.
   - Neurogenic incontinence occurs due to a lesion of the nervous system that causes a loss of sensation to void or a lack of bladder control.

a. **Etiology**
   - Weakened pelvic musculature from multiparity, obesity, trauma
   - Compression of urethra and bladder by
     • prostatic hypertrophy
     • fecal impaction

• have patient tighten anal sphincter (for about 10 seconds) as though holding in bowel movement, then relax, tighten vagina as though stopping urinary flow, then relax
• repeat procedure several times each hour
- Treat incontinent episodes in a matter-of-fact manner; do not chastise patient or overemphasize problem; reinforce teaching on how incontinent episodes can be prevented.
- Provide patient support for using assistive devices; help conceal them when in use.
- Ensure that toilet facilities are always readily available.
- Encourage patient to verbalize fears and concerns; encourage socialization and a normal life-style.
- Encourage patients to limit oral intake after dinner and to avoid alcohol, tea, and coffee.
- Teach self-catherization, if indicated, prior to discharge and provide patient with appropriate equipment; arrange a home health nursing referral as needed.

Table 6.3   Bladder Retraining

Purpose
  To reestablish partial to full control of bladder without retention, overflow, or infection.
Assessment
  General physical and mental condition
  Urinary tract function
  Cause, duration, and degree of incontinence
  Anticipated cooperation of patient and family
Preliminary Actions
  Keep a record of patient's voiding pattern: time, amount voided, fluid intake, and related factors.
  Note the amount of time between when patient goes to bed and first voiding episode to estimate how long patient can hold urine. Ensure that daytime toileting intervals do not exceed that time.
  Establish schedule of expected voiding times based on patient's individual incontinence record.
  Administer any prescribed diuretics early in the day
  Encourage up to 3000 cc fluid intake between 8 A.M. and 8 P.M. daily. Decrease, but do not discontinue, fluid intake after 8 P.M.
Voiding procedure
  Toilet patient approximately 30 minutes before expected voiding time.
  Encourage voiding by measures such as running water, tightening and relaxing pelvic muscles, rocking back and forth, and pouring a measured amount of warm water over the vulva or penis.
  Measure initial amount voided; then press on the lower abdomen over the bladder to express remaining urine (Credé's Method); measure this amount.
  Have patient practice Kegel exercises 4 times/day: alternate periods of contraction and relaxation of pubococcygeal muscles to develop improved muscle tone and sphincter control.

d. Evaluation
- Patient
  - remains dry and odor free.
  - uses toilet for voiding.
  - is free from accidents, impaired skin integrity.
  - maintains or improves self-concept
  - maintains or increases socialization

e. Possible Related Nursing Diagnoses
Potential for infection
Potential for injury
Self-care deficit: toileting
Impairment of skin integrity

Selected Health Problems Frequently Associated with the Nursing Diagnosis ALTERATION IN PATTERNS OF URINARY ELIMINATION

1. Urinary Tract Infections

a. Definition
Bacterial invasions of the bladder or kidney. This form of infection is common in the elderly due to the high prevalence of urinary retention, stasis, and calculi, and the decreased resistance to infection.

b. Etiology
- Obstructions of urinary flow
- Diabetes mellitus
- Prostatitis
- Senile vaginitis
- Frequent catheterizations
- Indwelling catheters
- Poor hygiene/poor wiping techniques in women (especially obese women)

c. Clinical Manifestations
- Frequency, urgency
- Burning in urethra
- Bladder, kidney, or suprapubic pain
- Elevated temperature
- Blood and/or pus in urine

d. **Multidisciplinary Approaches**
  - Analgesics, urinary antiseptics, antibiotics
  - Treat contributing cause

Additional Nursing Care That Can Be Incorporated into the Generic Care Plan

  - Encourage fluids (2000-2500 cc) daily, preferably before the evening meal to prevent concentrated urine.
  - Give cranberry or prune juice to acidify the urine.
  - Observe quality of urine (e.g., color or odor), the pattern and frequency of urinary elimination, and monitor I&O.
  - Prevent immobility, other sources of urinary stasis.
  - Use diapers and other alternatives to indwelling catheters if incontinence is a problem; the risk of urinary tract infection increases significantly in catheterized persons.
  - Use proper techniques to care for indwelling catheters (see Table 6.4).

2. Benign Prostatic Hypertrophy

a. **Definition**
  The enlargement of the prostate gland. It can lead to bladder outlet obstruction, urinary retention, and a distended bladder.

Table 6.4 Foley Catheter Care

Adhere to strict aseptic technique during catheterization, always using good handwashing technique.

Use the smallest diameter catheter possible.

Keep the system closed; replace only in case of contamination or loss of function; changing the system on a scheduled basis is not recommended.

Do not irrigate catheter unless obstruction occurs; prophylactic irrigation with antibiotics is not considered effective.

Collect urine specimens aseptically without violating closed system by cleansing area with alcohol, using sterile needle and syringe to withdraw specimen.

Keep urine from backflowing in catheter by always positioning bag below level of bladder.

Avoid kinks in catheter and other obstructions to urine flow.

Assure catheter is not accidentally removed or pulled.

Provide good hygienic care; special meatal care measures have not proven additional benefit.

Recognize signs of urinary tract infection (e.g., temperature elevation, cloudy urine, altered mental status).

Note: From "Urethral catheterization" by A. Kinney, M. Blount, & M. Dowell, 1980, *Geriatric Nursing 1*, pp. 256-263.

CHAPTER 7

ACTIVITY-EXERCISE
FUNCTIONAL HEALTH PATTERN

An active state is highly beneficial to older adults. Activity promotes lung expansion, circulation, digestion, elimination, muscle tone, bone strength, and other aspects of physical health. Healthy mental and social functioning is promoted, and in addition many of the elderly's health risks can be minimized by activity.

As advantageous as it is, activity is not an easy task for older adults. Stiff joints, shortness of breath, weak muscles, poor coordination, fatigue, and other disorders can make movement difficult. Other factors that restrict their social activity can be a limited budget or not having access to transportation. Inactivity can easily result from the common problems and changes the elderly face. Once inactive, the elderly are at risk for serious threats to their physical, mental, and social well-being, compounding other preexisting problems.

Activity is dependent on many physical and psychosocial factors including but not limited to well-functioning respiratory and cardiac systems; adequate nutrition; mobile, pain-free joints; freedom from chronic illness; and a desire to be active and participate in work or recreation with or without companionship. The elderly experience varying degrees of impairment in all these areas, whether the result of age-related changes or impairments caused by illness and disability.

Fostering maximum possible activity within the limitations of age and illness is a major focus of nursing.

GENERIC CARE PLAN FOR THE NURSING DIAGNOSIS
INEFFECTIVE AIRWAY CLEARANCE

1. General Information

Ineffective airway clearance is an actual or potential threat to the passage of air through the respiratory tract.

a. Etiology
- Decreased energy and fatigue
- Obstruction or infection of the trachea and bronchi
- Excess bronchial secretions
- Trauma
- Cognitive/perceptual impairment

b. Clinical Manifestations
- Abnormal breath sounds: rales, rhonchi
- Changes in rate and depth of respirations
- Tachypnea
- Cough
- Dyspnea, cyanosis
- Fever
  - respiratory infections are the second most common cause of temperature elevation in the elderly (behind urinary tract infection)
  - fever may be atypical
  - sudden shaking chills may be absent
  - high fever may not occur if normal body temperature is low

c. Multidisciplinary Approaches
- Chest x-ray
- Pulmonary function tests
- Sputum cultures/cytology
- Intermittent positive pressure breathing (IPPB)/oxygen therapy
- Postural drainage, suctioning
- Medications
  - antibiotics
  - steroids
  - cough preparations
  - bronchodilators
  - antipyretics

2. Nursing Process

a. Assessment
- Breath sounds
- Patient's color: skin, nailbeds, mucous membranes

- Vital signs
- Characteristics of cough
- Smoking and allergy history
- Sputum characteristics
- Posture
- Activity level
- Level of comfort
- Appetite changes

b. Goal

Patient will maintain/regain patent airway, optimal respirations.

c. Interventions

- Encourage expectoration and deep breathing every hour.
- Encourage fluid intake to 2,000 cc/day if not otherwise contraindicated.
- Humidify breathed air (use humidifier or place pan containing water on top of radiator or other heat source).
- Offer fluids hourly.
- Provide foods that are easily chewed and swallowed if patient is severely dyspneic.
- Offer frequent mouth care to increase patient comfort as necessary.
- Perform postural drainage if necessary, every 6 hours or as ordered.
- Monitor vital signs, color, and level of consciousness continuously to detect signs of hypoxia.
- Monitor effects of bronchodilators, relief of pain.

d. Evaluation

- Patient
  • has normal color.
  • is free from rales, rhonchi.
  • exhibits no shortness of breath, dyspnea.

e. Goal

Patient will be free from infection.

f. Interventions

- Monitor fever, sputum production.
- Encourage deep breathing, coughing every 2 hours.
- Provide and encourage use of tissues for disposal of expectorated matter.
- Ensure patient takes/receives prescribed antibiotics on time, and that entire prescription is delivered; assess for related complications.
- Teach patient early signs of respiratory infection (e.g., increased cough, increased production and/or viscosity of sputum, change

in sputum color to yellow, green, or gray; tightness in chest or dyspnea, fever).
  – Teach patient and family prevention techniques
    • avoidance of ill persons and large crowds
    • good breathing techniques
    • regular activity
    • no smoking
    • good nutrition
    • annual flu shot

g. Evaluation
  – Patient's
    • sputum production decreases.
    • vital signs are within normal limits, no fever.
  – Patient receives flu shot annually.

h. Possible Related Nursing Diagnoses
Activity intolerance
Alteration in nutrition: less than body requirements
Impaired gas exchange
Ineffective breathing pattern

GENERIC CARE PLAN FOR THE NURSING DIAGNOSIS
INEFFECTIVE BREATHING PATTERN

1. General Information

Ineffective breathing pattern is an actual or potential loss of adequate ventilation to meet individual needs.

a. Etiology
  – Decreased energy, fatigue
  – Pain, especially post-op
  – Decreased lung expansion
  – Tracheobronchial obstruction
  – Neuromuscular or musculoskeletal impairment

b. Clinical Manifestations
  – Dyspnea, shortness of breath
  – Tachypnea, fremitus
  – Abnormal arterial blood gas
  – Cyanosis, cough
  – Nasal flaring
  – Respiratory depth changes
  – Pursed-lip breathing and prolonged expiratory phase

- Increased anteroposterior diameter
- Use of accessory muscles
- Altered chest excursion

c. **Multidisciplinary Approaches**
   - Arterial blood gases (ABGs)
   - IPPB, oxygen
   - Bronchodilators
   - Occupational therapy

2. Nursing Process

a. **Assessment**
   - Type of breathing pattern (tachypnea, Cheyne-Stokes, etc.)
   - Results of lab studies, ABGs
   - Breath sounds
   - Pain, discomfort
   - Emotional response
   - See Ineffective Airway Clearance, page 122

b. **Goal**
   Patient will be able to demonstrate appropriate breathing techniques.

c. **Interventions**
   - Ask patient to take five deep breaths and evaluate quality of respirations; short breaths and movement of the shoulders indicate shallow breathing, contraction of the abdomen during inspiration indicates poor use of the diaphragm.
   - Teach the proper method of breathing
     • the abdomen, not the chest, should move
       * during inspiration abdomen should protrude and sink
       * during expiration abdomen should pull in and upward
     • have the patient monitor movement by placing one hand on the abdomen and one on the chest; only the hand on the abdomen should move during respiration.
   - Teach a rate of breathing that facilitates good air exchange
     • focus on forcing air out of the lungs because age-related changes can make expiration difficult
     • instruct patient to inhale to the count of 1 and exhale for 3 counts
     • have patient repeat exercises several times throughout the day; five repetitions of each exercise at each session are sufficient at first, but gradually increase this number
     • inform the patient that in addition to promoting respiratory activity, breathing exercises will also help to relieve tension and promote relaxation.

d. Evaluation
- Patient
  - practices breathing exercises at least 3 times daily.
  - exhibits no nasal flaring, use of accessory respiratory muscles.

e. Possible Related Nursing Diagnoses
Alteration in cerebral tissue perfusion
Alteration in nutrition: less than body requirements
Anxiety
Impaired gas exchange
Ineffective airway clearance

GENERIC CARE PLAN FOR THE NURSING DIAGNOSIS
IMPAIRED GAS EXCHANGE

1. General Information

Impaired gas exchange occurs when there is a decreased passage of gases (O_2, CO_2) between the alveoli of the lungs and the vascular system. Both hypoxia and excessive oxygen administration have serious implications for the older patient. High levels of oxygen can depress the respiratory center in the brain interfering with carbon dioxide elimination. Carbon dioxide retention results, leading to potentially fatal acidosis and carbon dioxide narcosis.

a. Etiology
- Altered oxygen supply
- Alveolar-capillary membrane changes
- Altered blood flow
- Altered oxygen-carrying capacity of blood

b. Clinical Manifestations
- Skin color changes, cyanosis
- Respiratory changes: increased respirations (may also be shallow and slow), air hunger, dyspnea, shortness of breath
- Behavioral changes: restlessness, anxiety, irritability, confusion, fatigue, drowsiness, altered level of consciousness
- Physical changes (late chronic signs): clubbing, "barrel" chest, 3-point stance
- Poor coordination, slurred speech, slowed reaction time
- Anorexia, weight loss
- Abnormal ABGs, decreased pO_2, increased pCO_2 (compensatory acidosis)

c. **Multidisciplinary Approaches**
    – Pulmonary function tests
    – ABGs
    – oxygen therapy
    – Bronchodilators, expectorants

2. Nursing Process

a. **Assessment**
    – Respirations, breath sounds
    – Skin color
    – Level of consciousness, mental status
    – Posture, coordination
    – Appetite

b. **Goals**
    Patient
    – will have adequate O_2/CO_2 exchange.
    – will be protected from complications related to oxygen therapy (CO_2 narcosis).

c. **Interventions**
    – Use the most effective method of oxygen administration
      • do not use a nasal catheter if the patient breathes through the mouth
      • avoid face masks if patient is emaciated
      • maintain level of oxygen administration between 2-3 liters/minute
      • check patient and equipment hourly (at least)
      • check blood gases results frequently.
    – Monitor for signs of CO_2 narcosis (decreased respirations, headache, flushing, altered level of consciousness, increased pO_2 and increased pCO_2).
    – Provide proper nursing care for nasal cannulas
      • keep humidifier filled with distilled water
      • ensure that the prongs stay in the nostrils
      • place gauze between tubing and skin surface over the ears; observe for signs of skin irritation and breakdown
      • lubricate lips and nose with water soluble (not petroleum-based) lubricant jelly
      • provide regular oral and nasal hygiene.
    – Monitor patient's vital signs, mental status, and skin color closely.
    – Post "Oxygen In Use—NO SMOKING" signs and enforce them.
    – Check oxygen equipment and setting hourly (at least).
    – Avoid use of alcohol or petroleum-based products in patient care.
    – Protect patient from static electricity and hazardous electrical appliances.

- Encourage activity as possible.
- Turn, cough, and deep breathe frequently.
- Evaluate effects of prescribed drugs and treatments.

d. Evaluation
- Patient
  - has pO_2 greater than 60 mm Hg.
  - has pCO_2 between 35-45 mm Hg.
  - has normal level of consciousness.
  - has good skin color.
  - breathes comfortably.
  - is free from impaired mucous membranes of nose and mouth.
  - receives oxygen according to safety guidelines.

e. Possible Related Nursing Diagnoses
  Activity intolerance
  Anxiety
  Ineffective airway clearance
  Ineffective breathing patterns
  Potential for injury
  Sleep-rest disturbance

Selected Health Problems Frequently Associated with the Nursing Diagnosis IMPAIRED GAS EXCHANGE

1. Chronic Obstructive Pulmonary Disease (Emphysema)

a. Definition
  A destructive lung condition in which the alveoli become distended and are fewer in number.

b. Etiology
- Cigarette smoking
- Air pollution
- Heredity (inherited deficiency in protein alpha 1 antitrypsin [A_1AT] leads to destruction of lung tissue)
- Age-related changes
- Allergy
- Infection
- Occupational disease
- Chronic bronchitis with repeated infection

c. **Clinical Manifestations**
   - Ruddy, pink complexion due to hypoxia caused by high blood CO_2 level
   - Expiratory difficulties
   - Dyspnea, shortness of breath, cough
   - Barrel chest (increase in anterior-posterior diameter)
   - Weakness, lethargy
   - Anorexia, weight loss

d. **Multidisciplinary Approaches**
   - Medications
     - bronchodilators
     - antibiotics
     - steroids
   - IPPB
   - Postural drainage

Additional Nursing Care That Can Be Incorporated into the Generic Care Plan

   - Keep oxygen administration at 2 liters/minute or below to avoid complications.
   - Determine impact of disease on functional ability
     - ask about ability to complete daily activities
     - review disease effect on appetite, sleep, energy, cognition, and other functional aspects
     - explore patient's and family's emotional reaction to disease; provide counseling and support.
   - Teach realities and care of disease (e.g., prophylactic use of antibiotics, breathing exercises, smoking cessation, recognition of complications).
   - Review safe use of medications and oxygen at home with the patient (see Table 7.1).
   - Instruct in identifying and avoiding environmental factors that can worsen condition (e.g., high humidity, pollution, extremes in temperature, cigarette smoke).

Table 7.1   Guidelines for Safe Home Use of Oxygen

- Remove fire hazards from environment.
- Instruct all persons in the home that smoking is not allowed; post no smoking signs.
- Teach family proper use of oxygen, including signs of complications.
- Secure the oxygen tank in a stand, in a safe location, at least 6 feet away from heat sources and electrical appliances.
- Keep oil, grease, alcohol, and other combustibles away from the area in which oxygen is used.
- Have a fire extinguisher readily available.
- Notify the local fire department that oxygen is in use at the patient's address.
- Close valves of tank when not in use.
- Post the prescribed setting on tank and reinforce the importance of not changing the setting.

2. Pneumonia (Bacterial/Viral)

a. Discussion

Pneumonia ranks with influenza as the fourth leading cause of death in older adults. The elderly are at particularly high risk because of their reduced respiratory activity, inability to remove secretions, decreased resistance, and presence of other conditions that reduce activity. The effects of this inflammation of the lung can be devastating. The most common form of pneumonia in the elderly is pneumococcal pneumonia. The pattern of onset varies. Pneumococcal and klebsiella pneumonias have a rapid onset with shaking and chills; staphylococcal pneumonia develops slowly with subtle signs.

b. Etiology

- Aspiration
- Chronic obstructive pulmonary disease
- Increased bronchial secretion
- Reduced ability to rid lungs of bacteria
- Upper respiratory infections
- Impaired respiration due to debilitation
- Postoperative weakness

c. Clinical Manifestations

- Fever
- Elevated pulse
- Rapid respiration
- Productive cough, pink to rust-colored mucus
- Cyanosis
- Confusion
- Consolidation (visible on chest x-ray)
- Elevated white blood cell count
- Anorexia

d. Multidisciplinary Approaches

- Oxygen therapy
- Medications
  • antibiotics (see Table 4.1)
  • analgesics (see Table 8.5)
  • antipyretics, cough preparations
- Sputum and blood cultures

Additional Nursing Care That Can Be Incorporated into the Generic Care Plan

- Observe for signs of complications (septicemia, paralytic ileus, atelectasis, lung abscess, congestive heart failure, dysrhythmias, delirium, meningitis).

- Provide comfort measures if feverish, such as increased fluids, dry bedlinens, gowns, cooling measures.
- Evaluate effects of antipyretics, analgesics.
- Monitor for signs of antibiotic hypersensitivity (see Table 4 1).
- Ensure antibiotic doses are given completely and on time to maintain appropriate blood levels.
- Maintain patient on bedrest; raise head of the bed.

3. Chronic Bronchitis

a. **Definition**
   A chronic inflammation of the bronchi with production of a large amount of sputum that results in bronchial obstruction. Symptoms develop gradually, often over years, and are most prevalent during cold weather.

b. **Etiology**
   - Infections of the respiratory tract (pneumonia, acute bronchitis)
   - Irritation of the bronchial tree (e.g., dusts, smoking)
   - Heredity

c. **Clinical Manifestations**
   - Recurrent productive cough
   - Frequent acute respiratory infections followed by a lingering cough
   - Production of thick sputum
   - Dyspnea
   - Wheezing

d. **Multidisciplinary Approaches**
   - Medications
     • antibiotics
     • bronchodilators
     • steroids
   - IPPB

Additional Nursing Care That Can Be Incorporated into the Generic Care Plan

- Identify and remove irritants in environment (e.g., dust, pets).
- Assist patient to stop smoking.
- Limit patient's exposure to cigarette smoke and other pollutants.
- Explore occupational factors that could contribute to respiratory problems.

4. Tuberculosis (TB)

a. Definition

A disease, most commonly affecting the lungs, caused by *Mycobacterium tuberculosis*. Elderly are at increased risk of developing TB from direct exposure, because of poor resistance to infection and presence of other diseases or debilitating conditions. Most cases of TB in the elderly are actually reactivations of earlier infections.

b. Etiology

- Infection with the tuberculosis bacillus
- Those at high risk include individuals receiving steroid therapy, those with history of TB, and residents of high density areas.

c. Clinical Manifestations

- Fatigue, weight loss
- Anorexia, cachexia
- Productive cough (often blood-tinged)
- Temperature (possible afternoon elevation)
- Night sweats may not occur due to decreased diaphoresis

d. Multidisciplinary Approaches

- Antitubercular medications: Izoniazid, PAS, Rifampin
- Laboratory tests (AFB, liver function tests)

Additional Nursing Care That Can Be Incorporated into the Generic Plan

- Administer medications as prescribed and observe for adverse reactions.
- Limit droplet spread by using tissues for secretions and instructing patient to cover mouth when sneezing or coughing.
- Follow good handwashing technique.
- Keep environment clean and well ventilated.
- Regularly screen elderly in institutional or group settings (day care programs, senior centers).
- Encourage good nutrition.
- Promote normal activities of daily living.
- Arrange for diagnostic testing and follow-up care such as chest x-ray, sputum cytology, gastric washings.

GENERIC CARE PLAN FOR THE NURSING DIAGNOSIS
ALTERATION IN CARDIAC OUTPUT: DECREASED

1. General Information

Decreased cardiac output is a reduction in the amount of blood pumped by the heart resulting in compromised cardiac function.

a. Etiology
- Hypertension, atherosclerosis
- Conduction defects of the heart
- Myocardial or valvular disease
- Congestive heart failure
- Chronic obstructive pulmonary disease
- Fluid and electrolyte imbalances
- Shock, sepsis, allergic responses
- Age-related changes: reduced myocardial efficiency; weaker contractile force; thick, more rigid valves; less elastic vessels; poor tolerance of tachycardia
- Increased tissue demand for oxygen: fever, chronic anemia, malnutrition, fluid and electrolyte imbalances

b. Clinical Manifestation
- Fatigue
- Dyspnea, rales
- Decreased peripheral pulses, jugular vein distention
- Orthopnea, shortness of breath, frothy sputum
- Dysrhythmias, ECG changes
- Altered level of consciousness
- Cyanosis, pallor of skin
- Edema

c. Multidisciplinary Approaches
- Hemodynamic monitoring
- Medications
  - diuretics (see Table 7.2)
  - antidysrhythmics (see Table 7.3)
  - cardiac glycosides (see Table 7.4)
- Corrective surgery
- Oxygen
- Dietary modifications

2. Nursing Process

a. Assessment
- Vital signs, color of skin
- Behavior changes (restlessness)
- Level of consciousness
- Quality of respirations, breath sounds
- Appetite and weight changes

b. Goal
Patient's
- cardiac workload will be reduced.
- cardiac output will be maximized.

Patient will be free from complications.

c. Interventions
- Monitor vital signs every 4 hours.
- Place the patient on bedrest.
  - elevate head of bed to reduce pulmonary venous congestion
  - encourage patient to turn, cough, and deep breathe hourly
  - implement passive exercises
  - be alert to problems arising from bedrest (e.g., pulmonary embolism, phlebothrombosis).
- Observe for and correct hypoxia.
- Monitor sleep and rest; explore use of sedation if necessary.
- Ensure quiet, stimulation-free environment; schedule activities to maximize sleep periods; avoid use of restraints if patient is confused.
- Carefully evaluate the effects and side effects of diuretic therapy (Table 7.2).
  - monitor intake and urinary output; the elderly are more susceptible to excessive diuresis when taking these drugs
  - weigh daily
  - review patient's history for conditions which would contraindicate or warrant special caution with diuretic administration (e.g., anuria, hepatic or renal disease)
  - administer diuretics in the morning to minimize nocturia
  - observe for signs of hypokalemia associated with diuretic therapy
    * include high potassium foods in diet to prevent toxicity (see Table 7.6)
    * administer potassium supplements if prescribed.
- Encourage increase in activity as soon as allowed.
- Offer explanations, reassurance and support to minimize anxiety.
- Be familiar with medications utilized to improve cardiac function (i.e., cardiac glycosides); see Table 7.4.
- Obtain baseline and regular reevaluations of ECG, pulse, blood pressure, electrolytes, serum creatinine, and BUN.

– Advise patient to
  • monitor pulse
  • wear an identification bracelet indicating the use of cardiac gly-
    cosides
  • store medications in tightly closed containers, away from light
  • be familiar with antidysrhythmic medications, interactions, side
    effects and dosage (see Table 7.3)

Table 7.2   Diuretics

Examples	Side Effects	Nursing Implications
Chlorothiazide (Diuril)	Headache, drowsiness, orthostatic hypotension, lethargy, confusion	Administer diuretics in the morning to minimize nocturia. Do not restrict fluids without explicit medical justification. Prevent side effects by
Hydrochlorothiazide (HydroDiuril)	Indigestion, nausea, vomiting, diarrhea	–monitoring blood pressure, I&O, vital signs, blood
Spironolactone (Aldactone)	Photosensitivity	composition
Furosemide (Lasix)	Fluid/electrolyte imbalances Aplastic anemia, agranulocytosis, leukopenia, thrombocytopenia Reduced glucose tolerance Ringing in the ears (associated with furosemide toxicity) Concurrent use of aminoglycoside antibiotics, some diuretics (ethacrynate sodium, furosemide) carry high risk of ototoxicity Simultaneous use of cortisone can cause excessive potassium depletion High risk of dysrhythmias when diuretics taken with digitalis preparations	–observing for specific concerns • hyponatremia (sodium below 125 mEq/liter) • low blood volume; reduced cardiac output –being alert to signs of dehydration: weakness, irritability, muscle cramps, fainting (may indicate fluid/ electrolyte imbalance, which increases the risk of digitalis toxicity and dysrhythmias) –encouraging consumption of potassium-rich foods (see Table 7.6) –observing for subtle indications of infection and hyperglycemia (especially in diabetic patients).

Interactions: all diuretics
Increases effect of antihypertensives.
Decreases effect of allopurinol, digitalis preparations, oral anticoagulants, oral antidiabetic drugs, insulin, probenecid.
Effects increased by barbiturates, analgesics, any drug that can lower blood pressure.
Effects decreased by cholestryamine (do not take less than 1 hour before diuretic), large quantities of aspirin.

Table 7.3   Antidysrhythmic Drugs

General Nursing Measures

Remove potential hazards from environment (e.g., chemicals that could be accidentally ingested, clutter on floors).
Listen carefully to expressed needs/problems.
Advise patient to change positions slowly, hold rails when climbing stairs.
Arrange for and monitor blood work.
Monitor nutritional status, I&O, vital signs.

Type	Characteristics	Nursing Implications
Atropine	Dry mouth, blurred vision, urinary retention, disorientation, constipation, tachycardia, heat stroke	Offer hard candies and good oral hygiene. Keep oriented.
Lidocaine	Confusion, slurred speech, depression, convulsions, bradycardia, tinnitus, blurred/ double vision, dizziness	Keep airway tongue depressor in patient's room.
Phenytoin	Thrombocytopenia, leukopenia, ataxia, slurred speech, double/ blurred vision, hyperglycemia	
Procainamide	Thrombocytopenia, hallucinations, confusion, bradycardia, anorexia, diarrhea, lupus erythematosus syndrome	Modify environment to avoid misperceptions. Arrange for treatment of joint pain, muscle aches, fever, rash and other symptoms related to lupus.
Propranolol	Lethargy, cold extremities, bradycardia, reduced white blood cell count, diarrhea, hypoglycemia	Protect from and observe for signs of infection. Maintain body warmth; ensure patient does not incur burns in effort to keep extremities warm (e.g., inappropriate use of hot water bottle or soaks).
Quinidine	Serious dysrhythmia, hemolytic anemia, thrombocytopenia, vertigo, confusion, cold sweat, restlessness, tinnitus, excessive salivation, diarrhea, abdominal pain, asthma	Promote orientation. Facilitate relaxation. Keep dry, guard against skin breakdown.

Interactions: all antidysrhythmics
Increase the effect of insulin, oral antidiabetic drugs, anticoagulants, antihypertensives, antropinelike drugs, barbiturates.
Decrease the effects of pilocarpine eye drops, cortisone, antihistamines, anti-inflammatory drugs, myasthenia gravis drugs.
Effects increased by atropinelike drugs (e.g., antidepressants, antiparkinsonism drugs, antipsychotics), aspirin, coumarin preparations, estrogen, phenytoin.
Effects decreased by vitamin C, alcohol.

Table 7.4   Cardiac Glycosides

Examples	Side Effects	Nursing Implications
Digoxin (Lanoxin) Digitalis Digitoxin (Crystodigin) Lanatoside C (Cediland D) Quabain (G-strophanthin)	Confusion, memory loss, personality change, apathy, irritability, agitation, hallucinations, delirium, depression, impaired color vision, headache, fatigue, drowsiness, dizziness, aphasia, ataxia, fainting, seizures Muscle pain and weakness, neuralgias, restlessness, nightmares, insomnia, anorexia, nausea, vomiting Bradycardia, congestive heart failure, premature ventricular contraction, premature atrial contraction, paroxysmal atrial tachycardia, atrial fibrillation, ventricular tachycardia or fibrillation, SA block, premature AV nodal contraction High serum levels of drug 2 ng/ml digoxin 35 ng/ml digoxin	Assure smaller doses are utilized; the half-life of cardiac glycosides is prolonged in the elderly. Therapeutic doses must be individually calculated. Monitor digoxin blood level and observe for signs of digitalis toxicity (classic symptoms of anorexia, nausea and vomiting do not occur as commonly among older persons; confusion and heart failure may be the first clue). Be aware if the patient has hypothyroidism as this further decreases drug tolerance; hyperthyroid patients may require larger doses to achieve described effects. Review patient's history for conditions contraindicating or requiring special caution in cardiac glycoside administration (e.g., anemia, rheumatic carditis, subacute bacterial endocarditis, hypocalcemia, antibiotic therapy). Review patient's history for conditions that increase the risk of toxicity (e.g., thyroid disease, severe cardiac disease, respiratory disease, reduced renal function, small body size, diuretic therapy, hypokalemia). Evaluate apical-radical pulse for a full minute prior to administration. Instruct patient and caretaker in procedure. Assess for side effect of gynecomastia (enlargement and/or sensitivity of male breast tissue). Observe closely for signs of toxicity and monitor pulse closely. If toxicity develops, discontinue drug, notify physician and monitor cardiac status.

(continued)

Table 7.4   Cardiac Glycosides (continued)

Examples	Side Effects	Nursing Implications
		Review all drugs administered for potential interactions. Avoid concurrent use of adrenalin and cardiac glycosides as serious toxicity can result.

Interactions: all cardiac glycosides
Effects increased by guanethidine, phenytoin, propranolol, quinidine; any drug that reduces gastric motility.
Effects decreased by antacids, cholestyramine, kaolin-pectin, laxatives, neomycin, phenobarbital, phenylbutazone, rifampin.
Serious toxicity can result when cardiac glycosides are taken with cortisone, diuretics, parenteral calcium, reserpine, thyroid preparations.

d. Evaluation
  – Patient
  • expresses reduction in fatigue.
  • maintains bedrest free from complications.
  • is free from complications related to drug therapy.
  – Patient's
  • breathing patterns improve.
  • color is normal.
  • intake and output is balanced.
  • weight remains stable or drops.
  • heart rate is lowered, strength of contractions is stronger.
  • dysrhythmias are controlled.

e. Goal
  Patient will experience normal heart rate and rhythm.

f. Interventions
  – Be familiar with antidysrhythmic medications and their contraindications (see Table 7.5).
  • atropine (anticholenergic; blocks parasympathetic nerve impulses)
  • lidocaine (treatment of choice in initial management of ventricular tachycardia)
  • phenytoin (similar action to procainamide and quinidine)
  • procainamide (similar action to quinidine; better tolerated)
  • propranolol (fewer side effects than most antidysrhythmics)
  • quinidine (reduces cardiac output; unpredictable effects; high risk of toxicity).
  – Assure that initially smaller doses are administered until response has been determined.

- Avoid combining antidysrhythmics (serious dysrhythmias can result); when combinations are administered, monitor closely.
- Review other medications patient is taking; avoid drugs with anticholinergic properties (e.g., antipsychotics, antidepressants, antiparkinsonism agents.
- Assure serum levels are below toxic levels and in therapeutic range
  • lidocaine: more than 5 mcg/ml
  • phenytoin: more than 20 mcg/ml
  • lanoxin: more than 2 ng/ml
  • procainamide: more than 8 mcg/ml
  • quinidine: more than 8 mcg/ml
- Monitor vital signs, ECG.
- Note if patient is taking antacids or other drugs that alkalize urine (alkaline pH increases cardiotoxicity).
- Observe for indications of increased intraocular pressure when atropine is administered to patients taking haloperidol.
- Monitor patients taking both procainamide and kanamycin, neomycin, or streptomycin for impaired breathing and muscle weakness.
- Review all drugs administered for potential interactions and side effects to assure medications are not administered to patients with conditions contraindicating their use.

g. **Evaluation**
   - Patient's dysrhythmias are controlled.
   - Patient is free from complications related to drug therapy.

Table 7.5 Contraindications to Antidysrhythmic Use

Example	Contraindications/Cautions	Comments
Atropine	Open-angle glaucoma, chronic bronchitis, prostate enlargement, myasthenia gravis, peptic ulcer	Antidote: physostigmine salicylate
Lidocaine	Used with caution in all elderly Renal/hepatic diseases, congestive heart failure, weight below 100 lb	
Procainamide	Severe peripheral artery disease, bronchospasms, hypoglycemia (or tendency), congestive heart failure, respiratory disease	Antagonists: isoproterenol, glucagon
Quinidine	Myasthenia gravis, hyperthyroidism, recent use of digitalis, congestive heart failure, impaired myocardial function	

h. **Possible Related Nursing Diagnoses**
Activity intolerance
Alteration in nutrition: less than body requirements
Alteration in tissue perfusion
Fluid volume excess
Impaired gas exchange
Knowledge deficit

Selected Health Problems Frequently Associated with the Nursing Diagnosis ALTERATION IN CARDIAC OUTPUT: DECREASED

1. Congestive Heart Failure

a. **Definition**
A cardiovascular state in which the heart is unable to pump an adequate amount of blood to meet the metabolic needs of the tissues. It is a chronic illness for most people.

Table 7.6   Potassium-rich Foods

All-bran cereals	Milk
Almonds	Molasses
Apricots	Nectarines
Asparagus	Orange juice
Bananas	Oysters
Bass	Peaches
Beans (navy and lima)	Peanuts
Beef	Peanut butter
Brussel sprouts	Peas
Cabbage	Peppers
Carrots	Perch
Chicken	Plums
Citrus fruits	Pork
Coconut	Prunes
Crackers (graham and rye)	Raisins
Dates	Salmon
Figs	Sardines
Flounder	Scallops
Haddock	Spinach
Halibut	Sweet potatoes
Lamb	Tomato juice
Lentils	Tuna
Liver (beef)	Turkey

Consider sodium and calorie restrictions when including these items in any patient's diet.

b. **Etiology**
    – Congenital heart disease
    – Rheumatic heart disease
    – Hypertension
    – Coronary heart disease
    – Cor pulmonale
    – Acute myocardial infarction
    – Pulmonary emboli, infection
    – Ectopic rhythm
    – Fluid overload

c. **Clinical Manifestations**
    – Shortness of breath
    – Fatigue, poor appetite
    – Dyspnea at rest (with advanced cardiac congestion)
    – Unbalanced intake and output
    – Mental status changes
    – Unexplained rapid weight gains
    – Left-sided failure
      • dyspnea on exertion
      • orthopnea
      • paroxysmal nocturnal dyspnea
      • cough (may be early clue)
      • nocturia
      • rales, wheezes
    – Right-sided failure
      • distended neck veins
      • symmetrical peripheral edema
      • hepatic enlargement and tenderness
      • abdominal distension
      • ascites
      • gastrointestinal discomfort

d. **Multidisciplinary Approaches**
    – X-ray, ECG, echocardiography
    – Oxygen
    – Drugs (diuretics, digitalis, vasodilators)

Additional Nursing Care That Can Be Incorporated into the Generic Care Plan

– Review the history of symptoms, onset, duration, precipitating factors.
– Assess the degree of pain, respiratory difficulty, nausea, fatigue, the presence of shock or impending shock (vital signs, heart tones and breath sounds, urinary output) and skin color.
– Educate patient to the changes required in diet (low-salt, high-potassium), exercise, and medication (see Table 7.6).

- Educate patient about the physiologic changes that have occurred and the need to make life-style changes.
- Instruct patient to weigh self daily to monitor weight loss and fluid retention.
- Teach patient how to do leg exercises in bed to prevent phlebothrombosis.
- Encourage frequent rest periods in presence of dyspnea, fatigue, pulse rate.
- Instruct patient to report symptoms such as swelling of ankles, feet, abdomen; loss of appetite; weight gain; shortness of breath.

2. Myocardial Infarction

a. Definition
The lack of blood supply to the myocardium, which results in tissue damage. Atypical signs and symptoms occur among the elderly and the first major clue may be confusion.

b. Etiology
- Atherosclerotic heart disease
- Hypertension
- Diabetes mellitus

c. Clinical Manifestations
- Pain not relieved by rest or nitrates possibly radiating to left arm, neck, and entire chest
- Dyspnea
- Drop in blood pressure
- Moist, pale skin
- Low-grade fever
- Nausea and vomiting
- Fluctuation in pulse rate (increase or decrease)

d. Multidisciplinary Approaches
- Continuous ECG
- Monitoring of cardiac enzymes, hemodynamic parameters, ABGs
- Medications
  - analgesics
  - nitroglycerine
  - antidysrhythmics
- Oxygen
- External or internal cardiac pacing

Additional Nursing Care That Can Be Incorporated into the Generic Care Plan
- Monitor vital signs, ECG
  - change in pulse can indicate dysrhythmias

- increased respirations may signify congestive heart failure or pulmonary edema
- a drop in blood pressure can be associated with shock.
- Administer oxygen as ordered to relieve hypoxic heart muscle; avoid high oxygen levels.
- Review arterial pH and pCO$_2$ levels (decreases can indicate metabolic acidosis).
- Monitor I&O carefully (anuria may occur).
- Be alert to dyspnea, coughing, and rales (signs of congestive heart failure).
- Note mental status (changes in mental function and restlessness can indicate inadequate cerebral circulation).
- Promote rest to minimize strain on heart; use a bedside commode, support limbs with armrests and foot stools.
- Encourage daily graded exercise and emphasize the importance of avoiding physical and emotional stress.
- Maintain a comfortable environmental temperature.
- Prevent constipation to avoid additional strain on heart (see page 99).
- Administer analgesics as prescribed and evaluate effects (see Table 8.5).
- Spend time with patient and encourage ventilation of concerns and feelings.
- Teach relaxation techniques (see page 232).
- Educate patient and family in realities of the illness, its care and restrictions, including dietary alterations, smoking cessation, sexual activity; explain probable necessary life-style changes after recovery; provide encouragement to make those changes.

GENERIC CARE PLAN FOR THE NURSING DIAGNOSIS
ALTERATION IN TISSUE PERFUSION: CARDIAC

1. General Information

Altered tissue perfusion involves a decrease in nutrition and respiration at the cellular level caused by a decrease in capillary blood supply. Critical areas of concern among the elderly include cardiac, cerebral, and peripheral perfusion.

a. Etiology
- Interruption of arterial or venous flow
- Cardiovascular disorders: atherosclerosis, arteriosclerotic heart/vascular disease, hypertension, congestive heart failure, pulmonary edema, hyper- or hypovolemia, aneurysms, varicosities
- Blood dyscrasias: anemia, thrombus, embolus; transfusion reaction

- Hypotension: septic shock, hypoglycemia, hyperglycemia, anaphylactic shock, hypovolemia

b. Clinical Manifestations
- Tachycardia, tachypnea
- Angina
- Dyspnea
- Altered mental status

c. Multidisciplinary Approaches
- Cardiovascular monitoring
- Dietary approaches
- Medications
  - antianginals (see Table 7.7)
  - antihypertensives (see Table 7.8)
  - anticoagulants (see Table 7.9)

2. Nursing Process

a. Assessment
- History of common precipitating factors, immediately preceding (i.e., the 5 "Es": *e*xercise, *e*ating, *e*xposure to cold, *e*xertion, *e*motions)
- ECG changes (see Table 7.10 and Fig. 7.1)
- Presence of risk factors (e.g., smoking, obesity, high stress, hypertension)
- Pain: degree, location, type, and duration

b. Goals
Patient
- will have improved cardiac muscle perfusion.
- will be free of related complications.
- will be able to state precipitating factors.
- will identify life-style changes necessary to improve condition.

c. Interventions
- Help patient identify factors precipitating attack and how to avoid them (prevention of attacks is important; recurrence over the years can cause myocardial fibrosis leading to myocardial weakness and congestive heart failure).
- Promote health practices that can aid in preventing attacks
  - weight reduction
  - improved stress management
  - proper diet
  - smoking cessation
  - moderate, regular exercise.

Table 7.7 Antianginal Drugs

Examples	Side Effects	Nursing Implications
Amyl nitrite (Vaporade)	Weakness, dizziness	Crush ampule in gauze or cloth; hold near nose for inhalation. Do not use near fire or cigarettes (flammable). Encourage patient to sit during administration. Expect effect to last approximately 8 minutes.
Nitroglycerin (Nitro-Bid)	Throbbing headache Dizziness Weakness Nausea, vomiting Skin rash	*Sublingual* Store properly to maintain potency −do not expose to light, heat, air −do not keep cotton in container −use non-metallic container. Expect rapid effect, less than 20 minutes duration. If possible, use *before* exertion that could bring on angina (e.g., sexual intercourse, exposure to temperature extremes). Elderly patients might have difficulty producing enough saliva to moisten tablet. Advise patient to sit or lie while administered because the elderly are more sensitive to the hypotensive effects of nitrates and can become dizzy and fall. Burning sensation indicates drug is potent. Repeat dose if necessary at 5- to 15-minute intervals; administer no more than three doses. Keep record of time taken and result. Instruct patient to seek medical assistance if three doses do not relieve attack. Renew prescription every 6 months. *Timed Release* Take at least 1 hour before, 2 hours after meals. Expect effect for 8−12 hours.

(continued)

Table 7.7   Antianginal Drugs (continued)

Examples	Side Effects	Nursing Implications
		Topical Apply to hairless area for uniform absorption. Rotate application sites. Thoroughly remove residue from previous applications. Expect action in 30 minutes, complete absorption in approximately 4 hours.

Interactions
Effects increased by atropinelike drugs, tricyclic antidepressants.
Effects decreased by cholinelike drugs (e.g., Mestinon, Prostigmin).
Propranolol can increase hypotensive effects of antianginals.

- Monitor for changes in mental status, visual, sensory/motor functioning, headaches, or dizziness.
- Observe for signs of electrolyte imbalances.
- Observe for sudden onset of cyanosis, respiratory distress, diaphoresis, anxiety, sudden onset of chest pain.
- Observe for ischemic signs from drug effects.
- Monitor vital signs and heart sounds on an ongoing basis, note changes in blood pressure; monitor postural blood pressures.
- Encourage patient to rest, and avoid activities that can increase the cardiac workload (e.g., straining when having a bowel movement).

d. Evaluation
- Patient
  - recognizes causative factors and changes activities accordingly.
  - is free from complications related to drug therapy.
  - stops smoking.
  - performs exercise regularly.

e. Possible Related Nursing Diagnoses
Activity intolerance
Alteration in health maintenance
Alteration in nutrition: more than body requirements
Fear/anxiety
Knowledge deficit
Sexual dysfunction

Table 7.8   Antihypertensive Drugs

Examples	Side Effects	Nursing Implications
Clonidine hydrochloride (similar to methyldopa, most effective when given with a diuretic) Guanethidine sulfate (one of the most potent antihypertensives available, reduces systolic blood pressure more than diastolic) Methyldopa (for sustained hypertension) Propranolol hydrochloride (slow reduction of blood pressure, therapeutic effect within one week, wide variation in individual plasma levels, higher incidence of adverse reactions in uremic persons, more drowsiness than with other antihypertensives) Reserpine (action can continue for as long as two weeks after discontinuation)	Orthostatic hypotension Nausea, vomiting, anorexia, GI disturbances Reduced white cell count (particularly with propranolol) and platelet count Impaired ejaculation Depression, confusion, nightmares, hallucinations, psychotic behavior (particularly with reserpine and propranolol) Bradycardia (particularly with reserpine) Hepatitis (particularly with methyldopa)	Monitor blood pressure. Advise patient to change positions slowly. Monitor nutritional status, I & O. Assure intake of adequate nutrients and fluids. Observe for signs of infection, unusual bruises, bleeding. Assure periodic blood work is evaluated. Advise patient that impaired ejaculation is related to therapy. Assess impact of sexual dysfunction on emotional well-being. Monitor mental status. Assess ability to participate in ADL and maintain safety and intervene as necessary. Reinforce reality. Monitor vital signs. Administer propranolol on a full stomach, reserpine with meals. Withdraw clonidine gradually to prevent rebound hypertension. Protect patient from cardiovascular effects of propranolol: patient with angina can develop myocardial infarction and die from sudden withdrawal, extremities may feel cold due to reflex vasoconstriction; signs of shock and hypoglycemia can be masked.

Interactions: all antihypertensives
Increase effects of barbiturates, insulin, oral antidiabetics, sedatives, thiazide diuretics, tolbutamide (by propranolol).
Decrease effects of antihistamines (by propranolol), anti-inflammatory drugs (by propranolol).
Effects increased by phenytoin (by propranolol), thiazide diuretics (by guanethidine).
Effects decreased by amphetamines, antihistamines, tricyclic antidepressants.
Concurrent use of guanethidine with digitalis preparations can gradually reduce the heart rate.

Table 7.9 Anticoagulant Drugs

Examples	Side Effects	Nursing Implications
Dicumarol Heparin (reduced effectiveness in elderly) Phenindrone (more harmful side effects than most anticoagulants) Warfarin (usually started at one-half the adult dose)	Bleeding; hemorrhage Unusual hair loss Itching Sores in mouth or throat	Observe for signs of blood loss: dizziness, headaches, bleeding gums or wounds, hemoptysis, vomiting coffee ground material, bloody or tarry stools, fever, chills, fatigue. Keep skin moist. Regularly examine oral cavity. Have vitamin K available (antidote). Monitor prothrombin times closely, a dosage adjustment may be necessary. Ensure patient is not taking salicylates (for arthritis, etc.). As 3 gm or more can promote hemorrhage, suggest acetaminophen as an alternative. Review dietary intake for vitamin K-rich foods which can inhibit anticoagulant action (e.g., turnip greens, broccoli, cabbage, liver, spinach).

Interactions: all anticoagulants
Increase effects of phenytoin, hypoglycemic agents.
Decrease effects of cholestyramine.
Effects increased by alcohol, allopurinol, antibiotics (broad spectrum), chloral hydrate, chlorpromazine, colchicine, ethacrynic acid, mineral oil, phenylbutazone, phenytoin, probenecid, reserpine, salicylates, steroids, thyroxine, tolbutamide, tricyclic antidepressants.
Effects decreased by antacids, barbiturates, chlorpromazine, rifampin, vitamin K.

Table 7.10   Common Cardiac Dysrhythmias

Dysrhythmia	Causes	ECG Changes	Medical Treatment
Premature ventricular contractions (PVC)	Myocardial infarction Heart disease Stress on normal hearts from effects of caffeine, smoking, or alcohol	Wide and irregular QRS complex	Some resolve without treatment. Xylocaine if heart rate is over 60 beats/minute. Atropine if heart rate is slow.
Premature atrial contractions (PAC)	Impulses originating outside sinus node Can occur in normal hearts	Abnormal P wave	Most resolve without treatment. Quinidine when treatment is indicated.
Paroxysmal atrial tachycardia (PAT)	Impulses originating outside sinus node Can occur in normal hearts	Abnormal P wave; perhaps indistinguishable from T wave of preceding beat Rate usually exceeds 100 beats/minute	Stimulate right carotid sinus by using a tongue depressor to initiate gagging for a few seconds. Metaraminol or propranolol may be given. Cardioversion (timed electric shock) used in serious cases.
Sinus tachycardia	Impulses travel at faster rate due to overexertion, anxiety, fever or other stress Can occur in normal hearts under stress	Rate exceeds 100 beats/minute	Eliminate underlying cause.
Sinus bradycardia	Digitalis or other drugs (secondary effect) Myocardial infarction Hearts conditioned by regular aerobic exercise	Rate less than 60 beats/minute	Most resolve without treatment. Atropine when treatment is indicated.
Atrial flutter	Arteriosclerotic heart disease Rheumatic heart disease	Rate less than 60 beats/minute	Most resolve without treatment. Atropine when treatment is indicated.
Atrial fibrillation	Arteriosclerotic heart disease Rheumatic heart disease	Irregular P waves Rapid rate	Digitalis (unless already taken). Cardioversion.

(continued)

Table 7.10   Common Cardiac Dysrhythmias (continued)

Dysrhythmia	Causes	ECG Changes	Medical Treatment
AV block	Arteriosclerotic heart disease Myocardial infarction	1st degree AV block: longer P-R interval 2nd degree AV block: some P waves occur without QRS complex 3rd degree AV block: no relationship between P waves and QRS complex; slow rate	1st degree: most resolve without treatment. 2nd degree: atropine isoproterenol pacemaker. 3rd degree: pacemaker; atropine or isoproterenol may be used until insertion.
Ventricular tachycardia	Myocardial infarction (secondary complication)	P waves independent of QRS complexes Wider QRS complex Rapid rate	Xylocaine. Cardioversion.
Ventricular fibrillation	Myocardial infarction	Every wave and complex irregular	Life support. Defibrillation (differs from cardioversion in that shock is not timed).

Selected Health Problem Frequently Associated with the Nursing Diagnosis ALTERATION IN TISSUE PERFUSION: CARDIAC

Angina Pectoris

a. **Definition**
A severe pain in the chest, often radiating from the left shoulder down the arm, resulting from ischemia of the heart muscle.

b. **Etiology**
    – Atherosclerotic heart disease (obstructs coronary blood flow)
    – Severe aortic stenosis or insufficiency
    – Anemia
    – Hyperthyroidism
    – Tachycardia
    – Precipitating factors
        • physical exertion

- cold weather
- sexual activity
- cigarette smoking
- strong emotions
- heavy meal

c. **Clinical Manifestations**
   - Pain
     - mild to severe (usually lasting 3-5 minutes)
     - located at middle or upper portion of sternum
     - radiates to neck, jaws, and shoulders
     - more diffuse in many older patients

Figure 7.1 Understanding the Electrocardiogram

NORMAL SINUS RHYTHM (NSR)

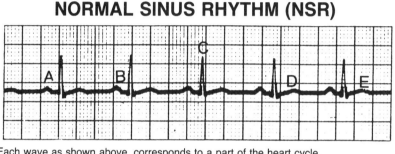

Each wave as shown above, corresponds to a part of the heart cycle.

A. P wave — Represents contraction of the atria. Normally does not exceed 3 mm (3 small squares) in height or .12 second (3 small squares) in width. A larger P wave indicates atrial enlargement.

B. P-R interval — Represents time between start of atrial contraction to start of ventricular contraction. Normally does not exceed .20 second (5 small squares) in width. Prolonged P-R interval indicates cardiac damage.

C. QRS complex — Represents contraction of the ventricles. Normally Q wave should not exceed .04 second (1 small square) in width or exceed 1/3 the height of the QRS complex. An enlarged Q wave indicates an old coronary occlusion. An enlarged R wave indicates ventricular enlargement; a smaller R wave occurs when the heart is compressed by fluid.

D. S-T segment — A segment longer than 8 squares indicates hypocalcemia; a segment shorter than 4 squares represents hypercalcemia. An elevation of the segment above the baseline indicates myocardial infarction or pericarditis; a depression of the segment indicates reduced oxygen supply to the heart muscle.

E. T wave — Represents ventricular recovery. Normally should not exceed 10 mm (10 small squares) in height. A flat wave indicates a reduced supply of oxygen to the heart muscle; an inverted wave indicates myocardial infarction. An elevated T wave indicates elevated serum potassium.

Note: From *Memory Bank for Critical Care* (2nd ed.), by G. Ervin, 1980, p.19. Baltimore: Williams & Wilkins.

- • difficult to detect and may be first clue
- • tight, strangling, vicelike feeling around chest
- – Apprehension
- – Weakness
- – Numbness in arms and hands

d. Multidisciplinary Approaches
- – Medication
  - • nitroglycerin
  - • vasodilators
  - • betablockers
  - • oxygen
- – Coronary artery bypass surgery
- – Dietary, exercise regimens

Additional Nursing Care That Can Be Incorporated into the Generic Care Plan

- – Assess the type of pain to determine if it is angina; anginal pain does not vary with breathing or body positions and is diffuse.
- – Administer oxygen and medications as ordered, observing effects.
- – Put patient in a comfortable position and give support in a calm manner.
- – Instruct patient how to take nitroglycerin properly
  - • keep in a tightly closed glass bottle
  - • place underneath the tongue and let it dissolve
  - • do not stand up quickly because of potential postural hypotension
  - • take again in 5 minutes if no pain relief.

GENERIC CARE PLAN FOR THE NURSING DIAGNOSIS
ALTERATION IN TISSUE PERFUSION: CEREBRAL

1. General Information

a. Etiology
- – Interruption of blood flow
- – Diabetes
- – Cardiovascular disorders
- – Aneurysm, arteriovenous malformations

b. Clinical Manifestations
- – Confusion, memory losses
- – Restlessness
- – Altered level of consciousness
- – Altered thought processes

c. **Multidisciplinary Approaches**
  − Cardiovascular monitoring
  − Medications

2. Nursing Process

a. **Assessment**
  − History of episodes of confusion/blackout duration, symptoms/ deficits exhibited, previous attacks
  − Vital signs, postural blood pressure, electrolyte imbalance
  − Reduced sensation: decreased ability to feel pain or pressure, numbness
  − Mental status changes: increased forgetfulness, periods of confusion, inability to recall own name, familiar objects or persons
  − Visual field limitations: blind spots, bumping into objects on a given side; homonymous hemianopsis: blindness in one-half of visual field, affects the same visual field in both eyes (patient may be unaware of the condition)
  − Swallowing problems: choking, feeling of knot in throat
  − Muscle weakness: drooping eyelid; drooling; asymmetry in strength, function, or appearance
  − Current medications
  − Predisposing medical conditions
  − Physical, mental, and social function prior to onset compared to present

b. **Goals**
  Patient
  − will achieve and maintain the highest level of functioning possible.
  − will be free from complications.

c. **Interventions**
  − Monitor vital signs and neurologic status.
  − Avoid situations that increase intracranial pressure (e.g., coughing, sneezing, straining, fever).
  − Give passive ROM every shift and have patient turn, cough, deep breathe every 2 hours.
  − Monitor administration of anticoagulants closely (see Table 7.9); observe closely patients who have congestive heart failure, indwelling catheters, or cardiac failure because their risk of bleeding is heightened.
  − Maintain and promote a good nutritional state; elderly patients with poor nutritional status have a higher risk of uncontrolled bleeding.
  − Adjust care to patient's particular needs
    • schedule longer periods of time for care activities
    • talk with patient during care activities

- do not assume patient doesn't understand
- keep patient informed of current events
- use simple, straightforward directions, one-step instructions
- provide clocks, calendars, and familiar possessions
- anticipate emotional lability and depression
- help family understand dynamics of condition and rehabilitation plans
- do not take patient's profanity or criticisms personally.
- Recognize demands of adapting to deficits
  - be aware that considerable emotional and physical energy is expended so patient may tire easily
  - allow frequent rest periods throughout the day
  - maintain a slow pace in activities.
- Implement procedures to prevent some of the more common complications (e.g., contractures, constipation, decubiti, trauma to affected side, edema in dangling limbs, falls, accidents, choking, sensory deprivation and isolation, fatigue, unnecessary dependency).

d. Evaluation
- Patient's
  - vital signs remain stable.
  - functional deficits are stabilized.
  - necessary rehabilitation is initiated.
- Patient is free from contractures, skin impairment, injury.

e. Possible Related Nursing Diagnoses
Alteration in patterns of urinary elimination: incontinence
Impaired physical mobility
Impaired verbal communication
Potential for injury
Self-care deficit
Sensory-perceptual alteration

Selected Health Problems Frequently Associated with the Nursing Diagnosis ALTERATION IN TISSUE PERFUSION: CEREBRAL

1. Transient Ischemic Attack (TIA)

a. Definition/Discussion
An impairment of cerebral blood flow that causes central nervous system dysfunction lasting several minutes to several hours. There

are no apparent residual effects nor any neurologic deficit between attacks. TIA is considered to be a warning signal and is part of the stroke syndrome. There can be a sudden onset of signs indicating interrupted cerebral circulation that usually last less than one day. Diabetes and coronary artery disease are contributing factors.

b. Etiology
- Atherosclerosis
- Emboli, plaques
- Blood vessel spasms
- Hypertension

c. Clinical Manifestations
- Falling
- Inability to speak or understand speech
- Double vision or unilateral blindness
- Amnesia
- Inability to recognize familiar persons or objects
- Numbness or complete loss of function in extremities

d. Multidisciplinary Approaches
- Anticoagulants, antiplatelet drugs
- Carotid endarterectomy
- Physical therapy

Additional Nursing Care That Can Be Incorporated into the Generic Care Plan

- Emphasize importance of adhering to treatment plan and seeking prompt medical care (TIA is a serious sign; risk of cerebrovascular accident increases with each TIA).
- Instruct in emergency actions to take when an attack occurs.
- Aid family in developing mechanism to monitor patient (e.g., daily phone call at mutually agreed-upon time).
- Teach safe use of prescribed medications and recognition of adverse reactions (see Table 7.9).
- Instruct patient to change positions slowly (e.g., sit on side of bed 2 minutes before standing).

2. Cerebrovascular Accident (CVA)

a. Definition
A severe, sudden decrease in cerebral circulation caused either by a thrombus (usual cause in the elderly) or a hemorrhage resulting in a cerebral infarct. CVA, also known as a stroke, is the most common neurologic cause of problems related to coordination and mobility. The chances of stroke are increased in the elderly and men are more

prone to strokes than women. Symptoms can appear suddenly and profoundly or slowly and subtly; will vary depending on area of brain involved.

b. **Etiology**
- Hypertension
- Atherosclerosis
- Cardiac disease
- Blood lipid abnormalities
- Impaired glucose tolerance
- Diabetes mellitus

c. **Clinical Manifestations**
- Paralysis
  • hemiplegia
  • quadriplegia
- Loss of visual field
- Spatial-perceptual deficits
- Incontinence
- Sensory loss
- Impaired memory and judgment
- Change in level of consciousness
- Difficulty swallowing
- Loss of control of emotions
- Speech and language alterations
- Anterior frontal lobe CVA
  • intact comprehension
  • altered speech
  • profanity used uncharacteristically and/or uncontrollably
  • altered sentence structure
  • impaired recognition of familiar objects
- Posterior frontal lobe CVA
  • comprehension lost
  • patient may make up words
  • groups words inappropriately

d. **Multidisciplinary Approaches**
- Medications
  • anticoagulants (if thrombus)
  • vasodilators
- Rehabilitation: physical, occupational, speech therapy

Additional Nursing Care That Can Be Incorporated into the Generic Care Plan

- Be aware of cognitive deficits associated with right and left lesions
  • right hemisphere lesion (left hemiplegia): no awareness of deficit(s), no depth perception, poor judgment, short attention span/easily dis-

tracted, inability to transfer learning, quick, impulsive movements, performance affected (not comprehension), not likely to regain pre-stroke capabilities
- left hemisphere lesion (right hemiplegia): aware of deficits; impaired ability to read, write, speak; repetitious actions, speech; slow, cautious movements; comprehension affected; prestroke function more easily restored.
- Review impact of illness and expected outcome with patient and family
  - current limitations and realistic expection of improvement
  - degree and duration of care required
  - most appropriate care setting
- Recognize new physical and emotional demands placed on family and care givers and offer support.
- Allow opportunities for ventilation of feelings; accept anger, depression, and other feelings as reactions to illness.
- Reinforce progress made and maintain a spirit of hope.
- Refer to the following nursing diagnoses for additional interventions
  - self-care deficit, page 182
  - impaired mobility, page 164
  - impaired verbal communication, page 203
  - grieving, page 266
  - sensory-perceptual alteration: visual, page 205
  - impairment of skin integrity, page 89
  - alteration in urinary elimination, page 112

GENERIC CARE PLAN FOR THE NURSING DIAGNOSIS
ALTERATION IN TISSUE PERFUSION: PERIPHERAL

1. General Information

a. Etiology
- Prolonged immobility or bedrest
- Obesity
- Thrombosis, emboli
- Hypothermia
- Contractures

b. Clinical Manifestations
- Claudication, flushing
- Change in skin color and temperature: cool, mottled, cyanotic, moist, absent/slow blanching, shiny
- Edema
- Slow healing of cuts and sores, tissue necrosis
- Altered blood pressure (high or low) diminished peripheral pulses
- Loss of sensory or motor function

c. **Multidisciplinary Approaches**
- Physical therapy, whirlpool
- Cardiovascular monitoring, Trendelenburg's test, venography
- Podiatry care
- Surgery: ligation and stripping of varicosities, bypass of occluded veins, tendon release
- Niacin

2. Nursing Process

a. **Assessment**
- Blood pressure, pulse pressure/deficit
- Pulse rate and quality: apical and all peripheral pulses
- Skin temperature, color, turgor, condition (especially legs and feet)
- Pain, cramps, numbness, tingling, burning
- Presence of visible, enlarged veins, edema
- History of predisposing conditions: hypertension, phlebitis, arteriosclerotic disease, diabetes mellitus
- Smoking history

b. **Goals**
Patient
- will experience improved peripheral circulation.
- will increase venous flow.
- will be free of injury to lower extremities and complications of decreased blood flow.

c. **Interventions**
- Advise patient to avoid constricting garments (e.g., garters), to wear support stockings that are put on before rising and taken off after returning to bed.
- Advise patient to reduce weight if called for and decrease saturated fats in diet.
- Encourage patient to stop smoking (decreases vasoconstriction and peripheral arterial spasms).
- Teach patient to avoid prolonged standing and crossing legs.
- Use foot cradle, sheepskin, heel protectors, lambs wool, and TED hose to protect the skin.
- Caution patient to rise slowly and carefully, allowing a few minutes of sitting before attempting to stand; provide assistance as necessary (blood pools in lower extremities, causing cerebral circulation to be reduced, and patient becomes dizzy upon rising).
- Encourage exercise (particularly walking) on a regular basis and increase amount as tolerated.
- Teach patient to avoid exposure to temperature extremes, and wear warm clothing.

- Instruct patient to monitor responses to walking and stop if s/he experiences pain, fatigue, dizziness, nausea.
- Have patient put extremity in a dependent position to improve arterial flow, and elevate extremity to increase venous blood flow.
- Teach patient how to reduce pressure points by range-of-motion exercises, uncrossing legs, changing positions.
- Ensure proper positioning to prevent contracted limbs.
- Protect legs and feet from cuts, bumps, and pressure; call the physician immediately if an injury occurs; skin is more susceptible to trauma, infection, and ulcerative lesions due to poor quality of circulation.
- Educate patient in principles of good foot health (see Table 5.5)
  - good fit, support, and comfort in footwear
  - avoid walking barefoot or in slippers for foot support and safety reasons
  - low, wide-based heels for safety
  - measure water temperature before washing or soaking feet (decreased sensations may prevent early detection that water is hot enough to cause a burn)
  - wash feet with soap and water and dry thoroughly, particularly between toes, apply lotions to prevent skin dryness
  - wear clean, well-fitting stockings, not tight enough to constrict or loose enough to wrinkle; avoid socks with dyes that bleed
  - keep toenails trimmed straight across, even with edge of toes; do not dig under nail or cut off skin (many elderly have visual or arthritic limitations; assess patient's need for assistance with cutting nails)
  - obtain professional care for corns and calluses
  - perform daily range-of-motion exercises for every joint
  - protect hands and feet from sun and cold.
- Give foot massages daily (a means to assess, stimulate circulation, provide exercise, promote relaxation) unless there is a thrombosis
  - clean and soak the feet
  - dry thoroughly
  - warm hands and apply lubricant to the palms
  - cradle the patient's foot in both hands for a few seconds
  - make circular motions with the thumb over the sole of the foot
  - roll knuckles over the sole
  - rotate and gently pull each toe
  - knead the heel and ankle
  - massage the heel firmly
  - allow the patient a period of relaxation afterwards.

d. Evaluation
  - Patient's
    - extremities are warm, color normal.
    - pedal pulses are equal and of good quality.

• feet remain clean with skin intact.
– Patient wears clean, well-fitting footwear.

e. **Possible Related Nursing Diagnoses**
Alteration in health maintenance
Alteration in nutrition
Noncompliance
Potential for injury
Sexual dysfunction

Selected Health Problems Frequently Associated with the Nursing Diagnosis ALTERATION IN TISSUE PERFUSION: PERIPHERAL

1. Hypertension

a. **Definition/Discussion**
A rise in systolic and diastolic blood pressure above the level judged normal for the individual. People over 50 years of age with a sustained blood pressure greater than 165/95 are considered to be hypertensive. Types of hypertension include
Primary (essential): No known cause and usually occurs between 30-50 years of age. 85% of all hypertension is primary.
Secondary: Cause is an underlying primary disease and usually develops before 30 or after 50 years of age.
Benign: A slow, progressive rise in blood pressure over 20 to 30 years of age.
Malignant (accelerated): An abrupt, severe rise in blood pressure (greater than 130 mm Hg diastolic); papilledema is present.

b. **Etiology**
– Age-related changes causing rigidity of the aorta
– Greater peripheral resistance
– Atherosclerosis
– Anemia
– Thyrotoxicosis
– Paget's disease
– Renovascular hypertension
– Stress
– Adrenal medullary tumor

c. **Clinical Manifestations**
– Asymptomatic
    • first clues to problem may be manifestations of underlying dis-

ease processes (e.g., transient ischemic attacks, mental status alterations associated with atherosclerosis).
- Blood pressure 165/95 or greater.

d. Multidisciplinary Approaches
- Medications: diuretics, antihypertensives
- Diet adjustments: low sodium, low fat
- Consultation for stress management

Additional Nursing Care That Can Be Incorporated into the Generic Care Plan

- Monitor vital signs, take blood pressure carefully on schedule as ordered (see Table 7.11).
- Note symptoms and function in relation to documented blood pressure.
- Ensure that antihypertensives are administered on time and consistently; monitor patient for expected effects or adverse effects (see Table 7.8).
- Be aware of and monitor the following risks of hypertensive therapy

Table 7.11   Obtaining an Accurate Blood Pressure Reading

Help the patient feel calm and comfortable.
- Avoid assessing blood pressure in extremely cold (or warm) environments (remember, the elderly are more sensitive to cold and can be uncomfortable in temperatures that do not bother nursing staff).
- Use a snug-fitting cuff of uniform compression; position the lower edge approximately 1″ above where stethoscope will be placed.
- Position artery used for the reading at the level of the patient's heart.
- Do not use a paralyzed limb to measure blood pressure.
- Palpate systolic blood pressure before auscultating
  −take the radial pulse (or popliteal if a leg reading is used) while the cuff is being inflated
  −note the point at which pulse is no longer palpable (systolic blood pressure).
- Reinflate the cuff approximately 20 mm Hg above the palpated systolic pressure; read with stethoscope as you slowly deflate the cuff.
- If several different readings are to be obtained
  −fully deflate cuff between each measurement
  −allow full circulation to return before retaking.
- If possible, take blood pressure in sitting, lying, and standing positions to detect significant postural changes.
- Record
  −blood pressure
  −extremity used
  −position of patient during reading.
- Pulse strength may vary in elderly persons, making the blood pressure difficult to obtain. In such cases readings may need to be estimated and should be noted as such on the chart.
- Take several readings to confirm blood pressure elevation; it may be useful to obtain a reading in the patient's home, on a different day, reducing stress from the strange environment and medical examination.

- persons with diabetes, reduced renal function, malnutrition, or on cardiac glycoside therapy have a higher risk of complications
- depression can be caused or intensified by antihypertensives
- antihypertensives can aggravate prostate problems
- orthostatic hypotension is more likely in patients with poor cerebral blood flow
- guanethidine sulfate must be discontinued several weeks prior to any anticipated surgery (vascular collapse, cardiac arrest can occur during anesthesia).
- Observe for episodes of hypotension; take blood pressure when person is supine and immediately again when person sits/stands upright.
- Maintain fluid and electrolyte balance.
- Educate patients and families about hypertensive disease and management
  - asymptomatic nature
  - need for effective stress management
  - importance of regular medication (even if symptoms are absent)
  - need for regular medical follow-up
  - management of low-sodium, high-potassium diet, low in calories for weight control
  - early recognition of complications such as congestive heart failure, myocardial infarction, changes in mental status, stroke, hypertensive retinopathy, renal disease.

2. Varicose Veins

a. Definition
Dilated elongated superficial veins most often seen in the legs, but can occur anywhere.

b. Etiology
- Age-related loss of tissue elasticity
- Prolonged standing
- Obesity
- Multiparity
- Hereditary weakness of vein wall
- Chronic constipation (rectal varicosities)

c. Clinical Manifestations
- Visibly enlarged discolored veins
- Leg cramps, aches
- Fatigue
- Edema

d. Multidisciplinary Approaches
- Support stockings
- Surgery: ligation and stripping of varicosities

Additional Nursing Care That Can Be Incorporated into the Generic Care Plan

- Teach preventive measures regarding avoiding prolonged sitting or standing, avoiding constrictive clothing, and obesity.
- Stress the importance of improving circulation and avoiding complications such as thrombophlebitis and ulceration.
- Instruct patient on proper use of support hose.

3. Stasis Ulcers of the Legs

a. Definition
Lesions that develop as a result of poor circulation. The ulcers usually occur on the ankles.

b. Etiology
- Chronic venous insufficiency
- Thrombophlebitis
- Incompetent valves of the veins

c. Clinical Manifestations
- Pain may or may not be present
- Arterial ischemic ulcers are usually more painful than venous ulcers
- Reddening of foot (may become pale when elevated)
- Leg edematous and cool to touch
- Poor pulse
- Skin changes (dermatitis)

d. Multidisciplinary Approaches
- Phlebography
- Compression bandages, Unna's boot
- Surgery: removal, skin grafts
- Medication: antibiotics

Additional Nursing Care That Can Be Incorporated into the Generic Care Plan

- Promote healing of ulcerated areas and keep free from infection, gangrene by
  • keeping extremity elevated and warm
  • keeping bed clothes off injured area
  • assisting with ulcer debridement as directed, maintaining strict aseptic technique
  • assessing effectiveness of ordered treatments (e.g., Elastoplast or Unna's paste boot)
  • monitoring for side effects of prescribed antibiotics

- assessing for and report any signs of cellulitis (e.g., redness, edema, pain).

GENERIC CARE PLAN FOR THE NURSING DIAGNOSIS
IMPAIRED PHYSICAL MOBILITY

1. General Information

Impaired physical mobility is a condition in which the person has some degree of difficulty or complete inability to move purposefully in the environment; may be imposed by medical order or the result of a physical impairment.

a. Etiology
- CVA, amputation
- Fractures, missing limb
- Arthritis
- Nervous system disorders
- Head injury
- Medical conditions requiring enforced bedrest
- Obesity

b. Clinical Manifestations
- Muscle weakness, paralysis
- Pain, inflammation of joints
- Decreased level of consciousness
- Incoordination, muscle twitching
- Muscle atrophy
- Contractures, deformities

c. Multidisciplinary Approaches
- Physical therapy and occupational therapy
- Medications
  - analgesics (see Table 8.5)
  - anti-inflammatory agents (see Table 7.12)
- Surgery (joint replacement, fixation)
- Dietary adjustment

2. Nursing Process

a. Assessment
- Ability to move arms and legs
- Range of motion in all joints
- Strength of grip, equality

Table 7.12 Anti-inflammatory Drugs

General Nursing Measures
Observe for indications of bleeding.
Ensure periodic blood work is ordered and evaluated.
Protect from hazards related to impaired hearing and vision, dizziness; assure
communication is understood.
Monitor vitals signs, mental status, intake and output, renal function.

Examples	*Contraindications*	*Side Effects*	*Nursing Implications*
Aspirin	GI disease, irritation Anticoagulant therapy	GI irritation Increased blood values: SGOT, SGPT, bilirubin, alkalie, phosphatase Impaired coagulation/ hemorrhage Bone marrow depression Liver, kidney damage	Vitamin C can increase drug's effects.
Adreno-corticosteroids	Cardiac, liver, or renal disease	Bone resorption, reduced formation of new bone Decreased glucose metabolism Fluid retention Increased risk of infection Aggravation of cataracts, glaucoma	Should be used with caution in the elderly due to high risk of serious side effects. Fracture potential is high so protect against injury. Monitor blood glucose, I&O, weight. Observe for signs of infection. Arrange for periodic ophthalmologic exams.
Cholchicine	Cardiac, liver, renal or GI disease	GI irritation Blood disorders	Preferred drug for treatment of gout. Observe for signs of GI bleeding.
Fenoprofen	Asthma	Hemorrhage Visual disturbances Impaired hearing, tinnitus Dizziness Renal failure (reversible)	Several weeks of therapy may be required for effects to be noted.
Gold salts	Systemic lupus erythematosus Uncontrolled diabetes Severe hypertension	Pruritus, dermatitis Stomatitis Thrombocytopenia Agranulocytosis Bradycardia Nephritis	Used to treat rheumatoid arthritis unresponsive to salicylate therapy. May take several months to a year

(continued)

Table 7.12   Anti-inflammatory Drugs (continued)

Examples	Contraindications	Side Effects	Nursing Implications
	Cardiac, liver, or renal disease	Hepatitis Corneal ulcers Anaphylactic shock	for full effects to be noted. Note complaints of metallic taste that could indicate stomatitis. Observe for skin irritation, itching; prevent skin breakdown.
Oxyphenbutazone	Anticoagulant therapy Blood disorders Temporal arteritis Dementia GI ulcers Glaucoma Cardiac, thyroid, hepatic, or renal disease	Bone marrow depression Hemolytic anemia Leukopenia Confusion Hypertension Visual disturbances Hearing impairment Hepatitis Renal failure Respiratory alkalosis Metabolic acidosis	
Tolmetin	Asthma Aspirin allergy	Hyperthermia Prolonged bleeding Dizziness Sodium retention Visual disturbances Renal failure (reversible)	

Interactions: all anti-inflammatories
Increase effects of oral anticoagulants, oral antidiabetics and insulin, penicillins, "sulfa" dugs.
Decrease effects of antihistamines (oxyphenbutazone), barbiturates (oxyphenbutazone), digitoxin (oxyphenbutazone), probenicid (aspirin), spirolactane (aspirin), tricyclic antidepressants (oxyphenbutazone).

- Level of consciousness
- Joint pain: quality, duration, schedule, relieving factors, current medications

b. Goals

Patient will be free from complications of immobility.
Patient's level of mobility will be increased.

c. Interventions

- Prevent immobility if possible; it takes an average of 7 days for the patient to regain the function lost during 1 day of bedrest (see Table 7.13).

- Position patient properly, maintain good body alignment
  - maintain body position as dictated by condition
  - change position frequently or at least every 2 hours
- Assess range of motion in every joint (see Table 7.14)
  - independent function
  - motion with assistance
  - note any pain experienced during joint movement
  - is joint motion adequate for everyday activity?
- Incorporate range-of-motion exercises into routine activities (e.g., bathing, turning, walking), rather than making the program an isolated entity.
- Encourage appropriate exercises for patient needs.
- When performing range-of-motion exercises for a patient
  - assure good body alignment
  - provide support above and below the joint being exercised
  - perform exercise slowly, smoothly, and gently, approximately five repetitions
  - do not force joint past point of resistance/pain
  - compare bilateral joint motion
  - record joint motion at start of program and its change with exercise.
- Use isometric, resistance, muscle-setting exercises if possible.
- Avoid positions that interfere with circulation (see Table 7.15).
- Ensure that patient turns, deep breathes, and coughs at least every 2 hours.
- Ensure adequate fluid intake, high-fiber diet if possible.

Table 7.13 Hazards of Immobility

Cardiovascular	*Musculoskeletal*
• Increased burden on heart	• Bone weakening
• Orthostatic hypotension	• Greater likelihood of bone fracture
• Thrombus formation	• Muscle atrophy
	• Contractures
Respiratory	*Urinary*
• Increased effort necessary for breathing	• Stones
• Poor gas exchange	• Urinary stasis
• Hypostatic pneumonia	• Urinary tract infection
Gastrointestinal	*Emotional*
• Decreased appetite	• Depression
• Constipation	• Anxiety
• Fecal impaction	• Preoccupation with illness
• Stress ulcers	• Feelings of helplessness and hopelessness
Skin	• Increased dependency
• Decubitus ulcers	• Exacerbation of latent neurosis psychosis
Neurologic	
• Sensory deprivation	

Table 7.14   Range-Of-Motion Exercises

- Range of motion: maximum joint mobility (varies in each body joint)
  • flexion (bending)
  • extension (straightening)
  • adduction (moving toward side of body)
  • abduction (moving away from side of body)
  • internal rotation (turning inward at ball and socket joint)
  • external rotation (turning outward at ball and socket joint)
  • circumduction (circular movement)
  • pronation (rotation down/toward the back)
  • supination (rotation up/toward the front)
  • inversion (turning in at other than a ball and socket joint)
  • eversion (turning out at other than a ball and socket joint)

- Purpose of exercises
  • maintain joint motion and muscle strength
  • maintain functional capacity
  • prevent contractures

- Types of exercise
  • active: patient performs independently
  • passive: nurse performs for patient
  • active with assistance: nurse and patient work together

- Be sure to provide adequate support for all involved joints when performing or assisting with range-of-motion exercises.

Joint	Normal Range of Motion	Exercise
Shoulder	Free straight arm motion from relaxed position at side, forward and overhead to a 160° angle	Flexion: With the patient supine, lift the arm above the head and return to original position.
	Free straight arm motion backward to a 30° angle with body	Extension: With patient prone, lift the arm and return to original position.
	Free straight arm motion laterally to a 160° angle	Abduction and adduction: With patient supine, move arm laterally toward head and return to original position.
Elbow	From full-arm extension, hand should swing back to touch the shoulder (160°)	Flexion and extension: Bend elbow and straighten to original position.
Wrist	From perpendicular with ground, wrist should rotate 90° to each side	Rotation: Hold the hand as if in a handshake (support above the wrist with the other hand) and rotate prone and supine.
	From parallel to ground, should flex downward 80°, upward 70°	Flexion and extension: Support above and below the wrist; move hand up and down.
	From parallel with ground, should move 10° (thumbward), 60° toward ulnar side	Flexion and extension: Support above and below the wrist; move hand laterally.

Table 7.14   Range-Of-Motion Exercises (continued)

Joint	Normal Range of Motion	Exercise
Thumb	Distal portion should bend 90° (right angle)	Flexion: Support thumb above and below the distal phalanx; flex.
	Proximal portion should bend 70°	Flexion and rotation: Support wrist and the area above the joint; bend and rotate thumb.
Finger	Distal phalanx should flex 90° (right angle with palm) and extend 30°	Flexion, extension, rotation: Support the wrist; using the other hand, simultaneously flex and extend all fingers (if a single finger has a limitation, do each one separately). Support the wrist and above the proximal phalanx; rotate each finger.
Hip	From supine position, rising toward the chin: 90° with the leg straight, 125° with the knee bent	Flexion and extension: Support behind ankle and knee; raise the leg straight up and return. Repeat with knee bent.
	From prone position: 5° backward extension	Extension: Support fronts of the knee and ankle; lift leg.
	From straight alignment with the body: abduction of 45°, adduction of 45°	Abduction and adduction: Support behind the ankle and knee; pull leg sideways, away from midline and across the other leg.
Knee	From prone position: 100° flexion	Flexion: With the patient in a prone position, support the front of the ankle, bend the knee toward the buttocks.
Ankle	Dorsiflexion (toward head) of 10°, plantar flexion (toward floor) of 40°	Flexion: Support ankle above and below the joint; flex in both directions.
	Inversion of 35°, eversion of 15°	Inversion, eversion, rotation: Support ankle above and below the joint; turn inward and outward, rotate.

- Use massage, lotion, or protective devices as needed to protect skin integrity.
- Ensure that patient has and knows to use equipment to summon help.
- If unconscious
  - protect eyes from drying, accidental injury
  - give mouth care every hour
  - provide head rolls, support feet
  - ensure patent airway; have suction equipment available.

d. **Evaluation**
  – Patient's
    • skin remains in good condition.
    • joints remain supple.
  – Patient is free from pneumonia, constipation, muscle wasting.

e. **Goals**
  Patient
  – will be safely mobile within the restrictions imposed.
  – will utilize mobility aids safely and properly.

f. **Interventions**
  – Encourage maximum use of mobility aids (see Table 7.16)
  – Teach proper technique for using specific aids
    • cane
      * use on unaffected side; advance when affected limb advances (i.e., if right leg is weak, the cane is held on the left, moved forward as right leg steps)
      * hold close to body; do not move ahead beyond toes of affected foot
      * all canes should have suction crutch tips to prevent slippage on floor
    • walker
      * when weight bearing is allowed, advance walker and step normally
      * when partial or no weight can be borne on one limb, thrust weight forward, *then* lift walker and replace all four legs on floor; always use two hands when transferring from chair or commode, back walker up to seat and use arms of chair/commode to assist in standing
    • crutches
      * tailor gait to patient's needs (consult physical therapist)

Table 7.15 Proper Positioning

Bed	Chair
No more than one pillow under head; do not flex neck.	Head straight; avoid bending or dangling.
Knees and hips straight: Use sandbags or pillows to prevent external hip rotation; do not put pillow behind knees or otherwise cause flexion.	Trunk upright, do not bend or curve.
	Arms and hands supported on armrest or tabletop; avoid dangling.
Angles flexed at 90° angle: Use footboard or pillows if necessary.	Hands flat; fingers open.
Arms abducted from body and straight with slight flexion.	Hips and knees flexed; feet flat on floor or footrest, ankles flexed at 90° angle. If legs are kept straight with a legrest, keep ankles flexed at 90° angle.
Hands flat; fingers open.	

* use good posture and pay particular attention to foot position on affected side—walking exclusively on ball of foot or toes can cause footdrop
* upstairs: step up with stronger foot; bring crutches to that step; raise affected foot
* downstairs: crutches to lower step; lower affected foot; follow with stronger foot
* general rule: stronger foot goes up first, down last

Table 7.16   Mobility Aids

Type	Characteristics	Fit
Cane	Assists balance by widening base of support; not intended for weight bearing	Length should approximate distance between greater trochanter and floor.
	Styles —regular (straight) cane • provides minimal assistance with balance – three- and four-point (quad) canes • broader base of support • more cumbersome	Elbow should be flexed slightly when cane rests 6 inches from side of foot.
Walker	Broader base of support; more stability than a cane Styles – pick-up • assists with weight bearing – rolling • pushed on wheels rather than lifted • reduces physical strain • often have seats which allow rest after several steps or propulsion from a sitting position	Height equivalent to distance between greater trochanter and floor. Elbows slightly flexed when grasping sides (of walker).
Wheelchair	Used when patient disability prohibits other walking aids Not a means of ambulation convenience or speed for patient or staff	Individually prescribed based on height; weight; required limb, head, trunk support; trunk, arm strength; self-propulsion capacity.
Crutches	Frequently difficult for the older person to use – inadequate upper body strength – arthritic hands – balance problems Not as stable as other mobility aids	Individually sized Length: equivalent to 2 inches below axilla to point on floor 6 inches in front of patient Hand bars – placement crucial; hands bear (or should bear) total weight – elbow should be flexed, wrist slightly hyperextended – axillar pressure can cause radial nerve paralysis.

> * eliminate obstacles
>   + waxed floors
>   + throw rugs
>   + extension cords
>   + uneven surfaces
> * wheelchair
>   * adjust environment: widen doorways and toilet stalls, plan a functional furniture layout with no rugs, low mirrors, telephones, drinking fountains and ramps
>   * lock chair; remove footrests for transfers; use special pads, cushions to reduce pressure damage; shift weight; reposition patient frequently
> – Consult physical therapist for guidance; teach patient how to fall and get up safely (fall toward affected side; use unaffected side to raise self).
> – Recognize progress and develop short-term goals to give patient a sense of accomplishment.

g. Evaluation
– Patient
  * uses aid(s) consistently and safely.
  * increases mobility daily.

h. Possible Related Nursing Diagnoses
Diversional activity deficit
Impaired skin integrity
Ineffective airway clearance
Potential for injury
Powerlessness

Selected Health Problems Frequently Associated with the Nursing Diagnosis IMPAIRED PHYSICAL MOBILITY

1. Osteoporosis

a. Definition
A metabolic disorder that causes a reduction in the mineral and protein matrix of bones resulting in diffuse reduction of bone density. It occurs in 25% of women and 20% of men over age 70.

b. Etiology
– Aging
– Deficiency of calcium and protein in diet

- Inactivity/immobility (causes high rate of bone resorption)
- Estrogen/androgen deficiency
- Hyperthyroidism
- Chronic disease

c. **Clinical Manifestations**
   - Progressive loss of bone mass
   - Weaker bones
   - Skeleton less dense
   - Spongelike appearance on x-ray
   - Kyphosis
   - Reduced height
   - Back pain and decreased spinal movement
   - Asymptomatic usually until a problem occurs such as a fracture or collapsed vertebrae

d. **Multidisciplinary Approaches**
   - Determine etiology (problems could actually be secondary to other disease [e.g. cancer])
   - Medications
     • estrogen
     • androgens
     • calcium, vitamin D
     • fluoride supplement
   - Treat fractures as needed

Additional Nursing Care That Can Be Incorporated into the Generic Care Plan

- Review diet for calcium and protein intake; adjust diet to meet requirement.
- Consult with physician and physical therapists regarding use of supportive appliances, bedboard.
- Avoid immobility; assist with range-of-motion exercises.
- Teach patient good body mechanics, ways to avoid strain.
- Protect limbs from fractures
  • support limbs when moving patient
  • handle with care
  • pad side rails
- Prevent contractures by proper positioning (see Table 7.15).
- Support patient in weight reduction program if indicated.
- Carefully monitor urine output (hypercalcemia can result in kidney stones).

2. Fractured Hip

a. **Definition**
   One of the most common orthopedic problems of the elderly, particularly older women. This fracture of the proximal end of the

femur can be intracapsular (femur broken inside joint) or extracapsular (femur broken outside joint). The complications arising from the hip fracture can predispose the elderly to considerable disability and deformity.

b. Etiology
  – Stress on joint
  – Falls
  – Osteoporosis

c. Clinical Manifestations
  – Affected extremity appears shorter, externally rotated, adducted
  – Pain
  – Inability to bear weight

d. Multidisciplinary Approaches
  – First x-ray may not show evidence of fractured hip
  – Traction
  – Surgery: internal fixation, prosthesis
  – Medications: analgesics
  – Physical and occupational therapy

Additional Nursing Care That Can Be Incorporated into the Generic Care Plan

  – Immobilize after fall has occurred and obtain x-ray immediately.
  – Control pain
    • administer analgesics as prescribed; monitor effectiveness
    • use caution and gentleness in moving extremity.
  – Begin rehabilitation as soon as possible
    • range-of-motion and isometric exercises
    • get out of bed as soon as possible
    • position body in proper alignment, prevent adduction and rotation of leg and hip flexion
    • encourage self-care.
  – Follow specific orders following surgical intervention.
  – Observe for and prevent complications
    • thrombophlebitis, embolism
    • contractures
    • skin breakdown
    • shock, hemorrhage
    • infection
    • hip dislocation, refracture.
  – Provide emotional support
    • patient may fear permanent disability, dependency; needs to understand new treatments that hasten recovery, rehabilitation advances

- may become discouraged during rehabilitative phase; set short-term goals, acknowledge minor achievements in recovery.
- Be aware of and support physical therapy plan.

3. Arthritis

a. Definition
An inflammation of the joints. There are three major classifications.

Osteoarthritis: Slowly progressing degenerative joint disease (middle and older age persons, more women than men).

Rheumatoid arthritis: Chronic inflammatory disease involving the body's connective tissue (occurs at any age but is more frequent in later years, more women than men). Insidious onset with progressive development of symptoms. There are periods of exacerbation and remission. (Elderly tend to have fewer remissive episodes.) Positive blood latex fixation, rheumatoid factor, and elevated white blood cell count in synovial fluid is present.

Gout: Metabolic disorder resulting in an excess of uric acid in the blood. Remission occurs between attacks. (90%-95% males over 50 years, 5%-10% postmenopausal women). There is an elevated serum uric acid, sedimentation rate, white blood cell count, and uric acid crystals in synovial fluid.

b. Etiology
- Osteoarthritis: aging, trauma to joints, obesity, heredity, inflammatory disease
- Rheumatoid arthritis: unknown; may be autoimmune, genetic, viral
- Gout: overproduction or underexcretion of uric acid that causes crystals of monosodium urate to be deposited in joint spaces; thiazide diuretics that may inhibit the excretion of uric acid; heredity

c. Clinical Manifestations
- Osteoarthritis
  - joint pain particularly on movement or weight bearing
  - may increase during changes of weather and after extended disuse
  - pain usually subsides with use
  - joint stiffness
  - altered posture and gait
  - sound (crepitation) with joint movement
  - bony growths (Heberden's nodes) on distal joints of affected fingers
- Rheumatoid arthritis
  - physiologic symptoms affecting small joints of hand
  - morning stiffness
  - joint pain, particularly on movement
  - swelling

- subcutaneous nodules may be present over bony prominences
- possible muscular atrophy of affected extremity
- systemic symptoms
- low-grade fever
- poor appetite
- weight loss
- anemia, fatigue, malaise
- Gout
  - severe joint pain that usually affects the great toe
  - often occurs at night
  - surrounding tissue will be red
  - swollen and painful
  - general malaise
  - signs of renal dysfunction

d. Multidisciplinary Approaches
- Medications
  - Anti-inflammatory drugs
  - Analgesics
- Comfort measures
  - Heat
  - Physical therapy
- Surgery (primarily for osteoarthritis)
  - Arthroplasty: replacement of joint with prosthetic appliance
  - Arthrodesis: fusion of bones
  - Osteoplasty: removal of deteriorated bone from joint
  - Osteotomy: excising bone to improve alignment
- Diet therapy
  - Low purine (gout)
  - Weight reduction

Additional Nursing Care That Can Be Incorporated into the Generic Care Plan

- Determine impact disease has on patient's ability to fulfill activities of daily living.
- Determine range of motion of all joints (see Table 7.14).
- Question about events that may trigger attacks such as stress, weather changes, specific foods.
- Discourage inactivity
  - perform range-of-motion exercises to the point of pain, but not beyond
  - involve patient in care
  - consult with physical therapist about strengthening exercises.
- Control pain
  - apply heat or cold (according to patient's response and physician advice)
  - use braces and splint during acute episodes and at night
  - prevent deformity

- Control inflammation
  - teach patient action, side-effects, dose, and administration of anti-inflammatory medications (see Table 7.12)
  - teach patient how to limit stress to joints, and avoid physical and emotional stress.
- Consult with occupational therapists about assistive devices to compensate for limited joint function.
- Review factors with patient that aggravate joints (e.g., joint strain, obesity, immobility).
- Provide support and counseling since awareness of progressive, disabling, deforming nature of disease often causes depression.
- Intervene promptly to prevent further erosion of self-care ability, discuss adjustments needed in life-style.
- Counsel patient to avoid "fad cures" and to discuss all forms of treatment with physician before implementing.

4. Parkinson's Disease

a. Definition
A progressive neurologic disorder characterized by muscle rigidity, akinesia, and involuntary tremor. There is no impairment of intellectual ability. The incidence increases with age.

b. Etiology
- Exact cause unknown
- Associated with cerebrovascular disease, viral encephalitis, and metallic poisoning

c. Clinical Manifestations
- Inability to control body movements (CNS impairment)
- Tremor (decreases with purposeful movement)
- Rigidity/slowness of movement
- Masklike expression
- Shuffling, rapid gait with trunk leaning forward
- Muscle weakness
- Drooling, difficulty swallowing
- Slow monotonous speech
- Increased appetite
- Emotional instability

d. Multidisciplinary Approaches
- Medications
  - antiparkinsonian
  - antihistamines
  - antidepressants
  - tranquilizers
- Physical, occupational, and speech therapy
- Possible surgical intervention (thalamotomy)

Additional Nursing Care That Can Be Incorporated into the Generic Care Plan

- Review impact of illness on daily living (e.g., feeding, swallowing, ambulation, hygiene, communication, toileting, safety).
- Adminster Levodopa or anticholinergics regularly to control symptoms.
- Eliminate pyridoxine (vitamin B_6) from diet when Levodopa administered (decreases effectiveness).
- Reinforce the need for regular medical follow-up; emphasize that although disease cannot be cured, its symptoms can be controlled or delayed with proper care.
- Expect emotional swings; explain to family and care givers that this is a normal part of the illness that the patient cannot control.
- Respect patient's intellectual status.
  - offer intellectually stimulating activities (e.g., reading, music) according to patient interests
  - speak to patient as an adult
  - be patient in allowing patient to express self
  - remind family and care givers of patient's real intellectual abilities.
- Offer emotional support; reassure patient and family that disease progresses slowly.
- Keep patient involved with social and recreational activities.
- Compensate for self-care deficits
  - teach alternate techniques for accomplishing tasks
  - obtain occupational therapy advice
  - introduce assistive devices and equipment
  - perform tasks that patient cannot
  - maintain maximum independence.
- Protect patient from hazards and complications such as choking and falls.
- Prevent contractures through range-of-motion exercises, massage, and proper positioning.
- See
  - Alteration in bowel elimination: constipation, page 99
  - Disturbance in self-concept, page 222
  - Impaired mobility, page 164
  - Impaired verbal communication, page 203

GENERIC CARE PLAN FOR THE NURSING DIAGNOSIS
ACTIVITY INTOLERANCE

1. General Information

Activity intolerance is a state in which the individual experiences an inability, physiologically or psychologically, to endure or tolerate an increase in activity.

a. **Etiology**
  – Any factor that causes fatigue
  • loss of endurance, age
  • depression, lack of motivation
  • sedentary life-style, bedrest
  • sensory overload or deprivation
  • sleep disturbance
  • treatments and diagnostic studies
  • equipment that requires strength (walkers, etc.)
  • pain, impaired motor function
  • lack of incentive
  – Any factor that compromises oxygen transport
  • cardiac: angina, dysrhythmias, congestive heart failure, myocardial infarction
  • respiratory: chronic obstructive pulmonary disease
  • circulatory: peripheral arterial disease, anemia
  – Chronic diseases: renal, hepatic, musculosketal, neurologic
  – Electrolyte imbalance
  – Hypovolemia
  – Malnourishment

b. **Clinical Manifestations**
  – Weakness or fatigue
  – Pallor or cyanosis
  – Confusion, vertigo
  – Inability to ambulate, turn in bed, perform self-care activities
  – Dyspnea, shortness of breath
  – Abnormal heart rate or blood pressure response to activity

c. **Multidisciplinary Approaches**
  – Rehabilitative therapy (physical, occupational)
  – Medication adjustment

2. Nursing Process

a. **Assessment**
  – Responses to activity (pre- and post-vital signs)
  – Ability to move, stand, turn without assistance
  – Causative factors (e.g., stress, psychologic, medications, disease process, life-style)
  – Determine current activity level and physical condition

b. **Goal**
  Patient will maintain or increase level of activity within individual limits of ability.

c. **Interventions**
  – Identify existing blocks to activity and plan to reduce or eliminate contributing factors.

- Teach patient and family the relationship between illness and inability to perform certain activities.
- Plan care to include rest periods to reduce fatigue; have patient participate in planning of self-care activities.
- Give pain medication as needed and promote comfort measures (see page 215).
- Protect patient from injuries by giving assistance when needed and do not allow patient to overdo.
- Encourage a plan of exercise that involves a gradual increase of activity as tolerated.
- Turn regularly and put all joints through range of motion at least three times a day if patient is immobile.
- Provide protein supplements to regular diet if necessary.
- Teach patient safety measures to prevent accidents and further injury (see Chapter 4, page 55).
- Increase patient's incentive by setting realistic goals; provide positive reinforcement and do things with the patient.

d. Evaluation
- Patient
  • is fatigue free.
  • tolerates an increase in activity.
  • implements alternate methods of activity.
  • balances activity with rest period.

e. Possible Related Nursing Diagnoses
Alteration in cardiac output: decreased
Alteration in comfort
Alteration in nutrition
Alteration in respiratory function
Fluid volume deficit/excess
Impaired gas exchange
Impaired physical mobility

GENERIC CARE PLAN FOR THE NURSING DIAGNOSIS
DIVERSIONAL ACTIVITY DEFICIT

1. General Information

Diversional activity deficit is the inability to occupy oneself in activities that pass time, entertain, or gratify. The individual experiences the environment as nonstimulating.

a. Etiology
- Physical limitations
- Long-term hospitalization

- Monotonous environment
- Lack of motivation or interest
- Retirement, "empty-nest" syndrome
- Loss of significant others

b. Clinical Manifestations
- Verbal reports of "nothing to do," "I feel useless"
- Yawning, inattentiveness
- Restlessness, boredom
- Withdrawn, hostile, lethargic behavior

c. Multidisciplinary Approaches
- Counseling
- Social groups

2. Nursing Process

a. Assessment
- Previous and current activity pattern
- Precipitating factors within environment
- Patient's ability to participate in activity (physical, mental, socio-economic)

b. Goal
Patient will be motivated to become involved in activities of interest that are personally fulfilling.

c. Interventions
- Reduce or eliminate causative factors
  - control pain
  - obtain mobility aids, transportation
- Offer activities that gave pleasure in the past.
- Encourage visitors, visitation of friends and family.
- Introduce to new activities; offer regularly.
- Increase sense of self-worth by providing positive reinforcement of skills.
- Encourage expression of feelings.

d. Evaluation
- Patient
  - identifies and discusses feelings.
  - participates in new or previously enjoyed activities.

e. Possible Related Nursing Diagnoses
Activity intolerance
Alteration in comfort
Anxiety

Disturbance in self-concept
Grieving
Impaired physical mobility
Powerlessness
Social isolation

GENERIC CARE PLAN FOR THE NURSING DIAGNOSIS
SELF-CARE DEFICIT

1. General Information

Self-care deficit occurs when a situation exists where the patient is unable to care for his/her own needs. The individual experiences a decreased ability to feed, bathe, dress, or toilet him or herself because of an impaired motor/cognitive function or emotional reason.

Ill, disabled patients will have differing degrees of overall independence/dependence in activities of daily living (ADL). An individual may function at different levels for different tasks. For example, a patient may be able to eat independently, bathe everything but the back, dress if helped with buttoning, walk and use a toilet independently, but will void on self unless reminded to go to the bathroom every 2 hours.

a. Etiology
   - Immobility, impaired physical functioning
   - Trauma or surgical procedures
   - Visual disorders
   - Pain, discomfort
   - Perceptual/cognitive impairment
   - Musculoskeletal disorders
   - Neuromuscular impairment
   - Decreased strength and endurance

b. Clinical Manifestations
   - Unable to feed self, cut food
   - Unable to wash body/body parts, obtain water, regulate water temperature
   - Unable to dress self, fasten clothing
   - Unable to groom self
   - Unable to get to a toilet/commode, flush it, or clean oneself properly
   - Verbal reports of "I can't . . ."

c. Multidisciplinary Approaches
   - Comprehensive physical and mental examination

- Physical, occupational therapy
- Mobility aids, assistive devices and adaptive equipment

2. Nursing Process

a. Assessment
- Functional capacity in feeding, bathing, dressing, grooming, and toileting (see Table 7.17)
- Causative factors (e.g., confusion, impaired sensory function, weakness, pain, missing limb, paralysis)

Table 7.17 Standards of Activities of Daily Living

ADL	Level I Independent	Level II Requires Mechanical Assistance	Level III Requires Human Assistance	Level IV Totally Dependent
Feeding	Able to eat without assistance	Needs special eating utensils	Needs food served and cut, packages opened, reminders to eat	Needs to be fed
Bathing	Able to get in and out of tub or shower and bathe all body parts	Needs grab bars, tub seats, adjusted faucet handles	Needs to be supported or lifted into tub or shower, back or other body part bathed	Needs complete bathing assistance
Dressing	Able to pick out appropriate garments and dress completely	Needs clothing and shoes modified with snaps or Velcro	Needs assistance with some garments and/or reminders of order to dress	Needs to be fully dressed
Continence	Able to completely control bowel and bladder elimination	Needs enemas, catheters	Periodically incontinent of urine or feces, needs to be reminded to toilet	Totally unable to control bowel or bladder elimination, catheterized
Toileting	Able to use toilet or bedpan and use proper related hygiene techniques	Needs bedside commode, bedpan, urinal	Needs assistance using commode or bedpan, wiping and cleansing after toileting	Unable to use toilet independently or clean self after elimination
Mobility	Able to walk and transfer from bed to chair	Needs cane, walker, crutch, wheelchair, brace, trapeze	Can walk, transfer, or use mobility aid with assistance	Totally unable to transfer, ambulate, or propel wheelchair

b. **Goal**
Patient will perform the activities of daily living within functional or mental limitations.

c. **Interventions**
   - Preserve and utilize existing ADL capacity to maximize patient independence.
   - Identify specific causes of ADL deficit; adapt nursing intervention accordingly (e.g., incontinence from mental impairment would require different approaches from those necessary if the patient has a neurogenic bladder).
   - Feeding: take food to patient and set up tray, cut foods, pour drinks, check in frequently to monitor amounts eaten and needs for assistance.
   - Bathing: lift in/out of tub, if necessary draw water and regulate temperature; bathe back, feet, legs; provide long handled wash-brush and soaped washcloth; remind to bathe specific areas and bathe completely.
   - Dressing: retrieve clothing from closet and select outfits for pa-tient; lay out clothing in appropriate order and encourage patient to dress self; provide special clothing (e.g., Velcro instead of but-tons) and special equipment (e.g., zipper aid) to ease the process of dressing; remind to dress; help with specific garments and/or dress patient completely if necessary
   - Toileting: provide bedside commode, bedpan, and urinal; assure easy access to bathroom and keep bathroom light on at night; assist in walking to bathroom or transfer to commode; remind patient to go to toilet and clean self after toileting, or help with cleaning; check for incontinence: provide sanitary pads, protective pants, or appliances as needed; provide change of clothing and assist patient to clean self after incontinence.
   - Mobility: See Impaired mobility page 164.

d. **Evaluation**
   - Patient
     • increases self-care capacity, meets ADL needs.
     • eliminates or compensates for deficits with adaptive devices or caregivers.
     • experiences no injury or complications.

e. **Possible Related Nursing Diagnoses**
Alteration in nutrition: less than body requirements
Disturbance in self-concept
Impaired physical mobility
Impaired skin integrity
Potential for injury

GENERIC CARE PLAN FOR THE NURSING DIAGNOSIS IMPAIRED HOME MAINTENANCE MANAGEMENT

1. General Information

Impaired home maintenance management occurs when an individual or family experiences difficulty in maintaining self or family in a safe home environment.

a. **Etiology**
   - Chronic debilitating disease
   - Injury to individual or family member
   - Insufficient finances
   - Cognitive, motor, sensory deficits
   - Inadequate support systems
   - Lack of knowledge

b. **Clinical Manifestations**
   - Verbal statements of patient or family having difficulty maintaining self-care at home
   - Poor hygienic practices
     • infections, infestations
     • unwashed linens, cookware, clothes
     • disorderly surroundings
   - Unavailable support system
   - Overtaxed family members
   - Financial crisis

c. **Multidisciplinary Approaches**
   - Comprehensive physical and mental evaluation
   - Counseling

2. Nursing Process

a. **Assessment**
   - Functional capacity, physical limitations
   - Mental status
   - Family system, support system
   - Resources
   - Housing layout, condition, size, safety

b. **Goal**
   The patient will be able to manage household independently or with help.

c. **Interventions**
   - Teach home maintenance management skills (e.g., food handling, disinfection, insect control).
   - Modify environment as needed (e.g., improved lighting, correction of plumbing or electrical problems).
   - Educate family to the availability of aids for home care (see Table 7.18).
   - Arrange for assistance through homemaker aide, volunteer, family member, home-delivered meals; social service agencies can offer guidance on available resources, financial aid.
   - Explore alternatives with patient and family (e.g., relocation, obtaining live-in companion or occasional housekeeper).
   - Discuss the possibility of a nursing home for impaired elderly.
   - Reassess self-care abilities on a regular basis
     - self-care capacity of patient or care giver may decline over time
     - repairs, security problems, new expenses may arise.

d. **Evaluation**
   - Patient functions adequately and safely at home.
   - Patient's level of self-care improves.

e. **Possible Related Nursing Diagnoses**
   Alteration in health maintenance
   Ineffective individual/family coping
   Potential for injury
   Self-care deficit

Table 7.18   Aids for Home Care*

Hospital bed
Trapeze bar
Overbed table
Hydraulic lift
Lift chair
Bedpan/urinal
Bedside commode
Bedding protectors/underpads
Protective undergarments/incontinence briefs
Bed-wetting alarm
Wheelchair/walker/cane
Grab bars, safety seats, nonslip strips for bathtub
Side arms, guard rails, and adjustable-height seats for toilets
Flotation cushions
Telephone amplifier and dial enlarger
Easy grip utensils
Vacuum-type feeding cup
Clothing with Velcro fasteners
Medical-emergency alarm systems

*Available through Sears Home Health Care Specialog or local medical supply stores.

GENERIC CARE PLAN FOR THE NURSING DIAGNOSIS
SLEEP PATTERN DISTURBANCE

1. General Information

Sleep pattern disturbance is a disruption of sleep time which causes the patient discomfort or interferes with the patient's desired life-style. Stage IV sleep (see Table 7.19) is decreased or absent in the aged. Their sleep is more often interrupted by nocturia, muscle cramps, and noise. After interruption, the patient requires more time to return to sleep. Less total sleep is required, but the frequency of naps increases.

a. Etiology
- Pain
- Stress, fear
- Insufficient daytime activity
- Nocturia
- Unfamiliar environment
- Interruptions

b. Clinical Manifestations
- Difficulty falling asleep
- Nocturia
- Sleeplessness, irritability
- Fatigue, yawning

Table 7.19 Stages of Sleep

Stage	Characteristics
I	Nodding, "dozing off"; sleeper awakens easily, will reach the next stage within minutes if left undisturbed.
II	Higher state of relaxation; some eye movement detectable through closed lids; sleep still broken easily.
III	Early phase of deep sleep: decreased heart rate, temperature, muscular relaxation; moderate stimulation required to awaken sleeper.
IV	Deep sleep: extreme relaxation, decreased vital signs and body movement; considerable stimulation required to awaken; deprivation can cause depression, apathy, and lethargy.
Rapid Eye Movement (REM) Sleep	Deepest sleep level: decreased tonus of head and neck muscles, increased, possibly irregular vital signs; EEG resembles Stage I; sleepers drift into REM from Stage IV about once every 90 minutes, 4-5 times each night, barring disruption by amphetamines, alcohol, barbiturates, or phenothiazine derivatives; deprivation can result in irritability, anxiety, acute psychotic episodes.

 – Nodding or dozing during the day
 – Awakening in the middle of the night
 – Complaints of wakefulness

c. **Multidisciplinary Approaches**
 – Treat underlying problem (e.g. cause of pain, urinary tract infection)
 – Medications (analgesics, sedatives)

2. Nursing Process

a. **Assessment**
 – Sleep history, usual bedtime
 – Sleep inducers used
 – Environmental preferences (e.g., temperature, lights, noise)
 – Number of trips to bathroom during night
 – Awakening time

b. **Goal**
Patient will be able to sleep 6-8 hours nightly uninterrupted.

c. **Interventions**
 – Accommodate patient's unique sleep habits by offering snacks, leaving radio playing, and providing extra blankets.
 – Assist patient in nonmedical means of bedtime relaxation such as baths, backrubs, warm milk, passive exercise.
 – Encourage activities during the day that promote sleep such as exercise, ventilation of feelings, proper diet, sensible medication and treatment schedules.
 – Avoid interruptions when patient is falling asleep (e.g., keep noise level down, do not flash lights, avoid bumping patient's bed).
 – Observe patient's sleep for frequent periods of awakening, breathing problems, and restlessness.
 – Discuss with patient possible underlying fears, conflicts and unresolved problems that may contribute to sleeplessness.
 – Avoid performing procedures unnecessarily during the night.
 – When hypnotics are absolutely necessary, use those least disruptive to the normal sleep cycle (e.g., flurazepam, chloral hydrate, diazepam, chlordiazepoxide).

d. **Evaluation**
 – Patient
   • reports adequate rest.
   • uses hypnotics appropriately.

e. **Possible Related Nursing Diagnoses**
Activity intolerance
Alteration in comfort: pain

Anxiety
Diversional activity deficit

References

Ancoli-Israel, S. (1981). Sleep apnea and myochonics in a senior population. *Sleep, 4,* 340.
Bahr, R. (1983). Sleep-wake patterns in the aged. *Journal of Gerontological Nursing,9*(10), 534-537, 540-541.
Spiegel, R. (1981). *Sleep and sleeplessness in advanced age.* New York: S.P. Medical and Scientific Books.

Cardiovascular Problems
Coyle, J., & Basta, L. (1983). Unstable angina pectoris. *Geriatrics, 38*(9), 79-92.
Curb, J. (1985). Detection and treatment of hypertension in older individuals. *American Journal of Epidemiology, 121*(3), 371-376.
Deckert, J., & Hom, R. (1983). Cardiovascular disease in the elderly: Diagnostic dilemmas. *Geriatrics, 38*(2), 48-52.
Hitzhusen, J. (1984). The elderly heart: Special signs and symptoms to watch for. *Geriatrics, 39*(6), 38-51.
Moss, A. (1983). Diagnosis and management of heart disease in the elderly. In W. Reichel (Ed.), *Clinical aspects of aging* (2nd ed.). Baltimore: Williams & Wilkins.
Spittell, J. (1983). Diagnosis and management of leg ulcer. *Geriatrics, 38*(6), 57-68.
Vidt, D. (1984). Treatment of hypertensive emergencies in the elderly. *Geriatrics, 39*(2), 55-68.
Webb, C., Horowitz, L., & Segal, B. (1984). Sudden cardiac death: An approach to management. *Geriatrics, 39*(4), 49-61.
Wright, J. (1983). Cardiovascular and pulmonary pathology of the aged. In W. Reichel (Ed.). *Clinical aspects of aging* (2nd ed.). Baltimore: Williams & Wilkins.
Zoler, M. (1984). MI: Recent insights—and new treatments? *Geriatrics, 39*(5), 123-136.

Orthopedic Problems
Albert, S., & Johnigen, D. (1983). Common foot disorders among the elderly. *Geriatrics, 38*(6), 42-55.
Cohen, B. (1984). Geriatric rehabilitation. *American Family Physician, 30*(1), 133-137.
Freehafer, A. (1983). Injuries to the skeletal system of older persons. In W. Reichel (Ed.), *Clinical aspects of aging* (2nd ed.). Baltimore: Williams & Wilkins.
Grob, D. (1983). Prevalent joint disease in older persons. In W. Reichel (Ed.). *Clinical aspects of aging* (2nd ed.). Baltimore: Williams & Wilkins.
Lane, J., Vigorita, V., & Falls, M. (1984). Osteoporosis: Current diagnosis and treatment. *Geriatrics, 39*(4), 40-48.
Levine, A. (1984). The elderly amputee. *American Family Physician, 29*(5), 177-182.
Mokowitz, R. (1983). Arthritis in the elderly: Some observations. *Geriatrics, 39*(10), 41.
Ringel, S., & Simon, D. (1983). Practical management of neuromuscular disease in the elderly. *Geriatrics, 38*(6), 86-92.
Stevens, M. (1983). Rheumatic disease: An overview of geriatic problems. *Geriatrics, 38*(10), 66-78.

Rehabilitation
Hunt, T. (1978). Rehabilitation of the elderly. In W. Reichel (Ed.), *The geriatric patient.* New York: HP Publishing.
Lonnerbald, L. (1984). Exercises to promote independent living in older patients. *Geriatrics, 39*(2), 93-101.
Sine, R., Holcomb, J., Roush, R., Liss, S., & Wilson, G. (1981). *Basic rehabilitation techniques.* Rockville, MD: Aspen.
Stevenson, J., & Gray, P. (1981). Rehabilitation for long term residents. *Geriatric Nursing, 2*(2), 127-131.

Stryker, R. (1979). *Rehabilitative aspects of acute and chronic nursing care* (2nd ed.). Philadelphia: Saunders.
Urosevick, P. (1982). *Coping with neurologic disorders. Nursing photobook.* Springhouse, PA: Nursing 82 Books, Intermed Communications.
Wolcott, L., (1983). Rehabilitation and the aged. In W. Reichel (Ed.), *Clinical aspects of aging* (2nd ed.). Baltimore: Williams & Wilkins.

Respiratory Problems
Acee, S. (1984). Helping patients breathe more easily. *Geriatric Nursing, 5*(6), 230-233.
Mostow, S. (1983). Infectious complications in the elderly COPD patient. *Geriatrics, 38*(10), 42-49.
Petty, T. (1983). Respiratory disease. In F. Steinberg (Ed.), *Care of the geriatric patient* (6th ed.). St. Louis: Mosby.
Reichel, J. (1983). Pulmonary problems in the elderly. In W. Reichel (Ed.), *Clinical aspects of aging* (2nd ed.). Baltimore: Williams & Wilkins.

CHAPTER 8

COGNITIVE-PERCEPTUAL
FUNCTIONAL HEALTH PATTERN

A ppropriate and effective interaction with the elements of one's environment is dependent on adequate cognitive and perceptual processes. Through perceptual processes the body uses its sensory organs to receive and carry messages from the external world. Cognitive processes then interpret those messages, using information retrieved from the memory.

With age, a variety of sensory changes can cause misperception of one's world; such changes include

- poorer vision: decreased visual acuity, narrowed visual field, slower light to dark adaptation, yellowing of the lens, distorted depth perception
- hearing loss: less capacity to hear high frequencies, increased auditory reaction time
- less taste sensitivity
- diminished olfaction
- increased threshold for pain and touch
- altered proprioception

These changes can distort the messages received by the body. Although intellectual function normally is not lost with age, poorer short-term memory and slower learning of new information can influence cognitive function.

In addition to the impact of age-related alterations in cognitive and perceptual processes, many of the diseases that are highly prevalent in the elderly affect the input and processing of information. Such conditions could include depression, anxiety, cancer, arthritis, peripheral vascular disease, cerebrovascular accident, cataracts, and neuropathies. In turn, a variety of physical, emotional, and social risks can develop from altered cognitive-perceptual processes. Promotion of optimum information processing and protection from risks associated with altered processing are crucial when working with the aged.

Patient education is important in nursing care to develop patient awareness of the realities of normal aging, health maintenance practices, disease management, safe medication use, the use of special equipment, and potential new behaviors.

Educating patients saves nursing time by enabling them to assume more self-care responsibility. Understanding enhances compliance with nursing instructions and helps prevent problems and complications. Being informed gives people a positive outlook on care and the patient will be less anxious and fearful when knowing what to expect. Patients are more apt to comply with medical regimens if they don't have to ask for and assemble fragments of information from different sources.

GENERIC CARE PLAN FOR THE NURSING DIAGNOSIS
ALTERATION IN THOUGHT PROCESSES

1. General Information

Alteration in thought processes occurs when there is a disruption in mental activities such as conscious thought, reality orientation, problem solving, judgment, and comprehension related to personality and mental disorders.

Elderly people are at high risk of experiencing confusion, a mental state in which reactions to environmental stimuli are inappropriate. The individual may appear bewildered, perplexed, or disoriented. Acute confusional states are usually abrupt in onset and reversible with appropriate treatment of the underlying cause. Acute confusional states differ from the progressive impairment of the intellect known as *dementia*, chronic organic brain syndrome, which is irreversible.

a. Etiology
- Sleep deprivation
- Psychologic conflicts, depression
- Drugs (barbiturates, anesthetic)
- Substance abuse (alcohol, drugs)
- Emotional trauma
- Environmental changes (hospitalization, relocation)
- Head injuries, brain tumors
- Metabolic disturbances
- Nutritional deficiencies, fluid and electrolyte imbalance
- Infections
- Conditions causing inadequate cerebral oxygenation (chronic obstructive pulmonary disease, hypotension)

b. Clinical Manifestations
- Inaccurate interpretation of environment
- Altered attention span, distractible

- Disorientation to time, person, place, circumstances
- Decreased ability to grasp ideas
- Changes in remote, recent, or immediate memory
- Impaired ability to make decisions, reason, calculate, conceptualize
- Hallucinations, delusions, ideas of reference
- Altered sleep patterns

c. Multidisciplinary Approaches
- Medication (antipsychotics) (see Table 8.1)
- Psychotherapy
- Recreational, activity, social services

2. Nursing Process

a. Assessment
- Mental status exam
- Extent of impairment in orientation, memory, thinking ability, attention span
- Changes in behavior, speech
- History of problem, how long it has existed, normal behavior
- Potential causative/contributing factors: drug use, dietary habits, presence of infections, sensory deprivation, stress

b. Goals
Patient
- will have maximum reality orientation.
- will be free from injuries.

c. Interventions
- Assist in eliminating or minimizing underlying cause (e.g., correction of fluid and electrolyte imbalance, discontinuation of drug, improvement of nutritional status).
- Be aware that confusion and restlessness may be worse at night; monitor patient carefully to avoid injuries.
- Promote reality orientation (see Table 8.2)
  • clarify misperceptions
  • offer orientation to person, place, and time throughout the day
  • use memory aids and simple one-step instructions
  • use clocks and calendars
  • do not support or ridicule delusions.
- Assist with decision making.
- Assure medications are administered appropriately; elicit help from family member or friend if necessary.
- Monitor nutritional status.
- Evaluate self-care capabilities and compensate for deficits.
- Prevent violent acts directed at self or others.
- Avoid overstimulation

Table 8.1 Antipsychotic Drugs

Example	Common Side Effects	Nursing Implications
Phenothiazine derivatives (chlorpromazine) Thioxanthene derivatives Butyrophenones (haloperidol) Indole derivatives (molindone)	Extrapyramidal symptoms −Reversible: reduced muscle movement/rigidity, weakness/numbness, masklike expression, monotonous speech, stooped posture, tremor, pill-rolling, drooling, heat intolerance, restlessness/insomnia, lost coordination tongue, neck, face −Irreversible: tardive dyskinesia (exaggerated motion of a single muscle group, often the tongue, mouth, face) Drowsiness, dizziness, lethargy Postural hypertension Photosensitivity	Explain unavoidable side effects; caution against −consuming alcohol, other CNS depressants −driving or operating machinery. Teach how to minimize adverse effects −rise slowly to avoid dizziness −use sunglasses, other sunscreening measures −suck on hard candy or mints −not to allow drugs to touch skin or clothing −consume adequate fluids, bulk Prepare male patients for possible sexual difficulties. Monitor vital signs, especially after giving Thorazine IM. Ensure periodic ophthalmic evaluation. Check bowel and bladder elimination. Keep I&O record if necessary. Monitor weight/prevent obesity. Obtain baseline CBC, liver function tests. Note signs of infection (e.g., fever, sore throat, cellulitis) that indicate development of blood dyscrasias. Consult physician regarding use of antiparkinsonism drugs to control extrapyramidal symptoms. Keep a flow chart/log of patient behavior evaluating medication effectiveness. Protect medication from sunlight; keep containers tightly closed. Protect patient from sun when taking Thorazine.

Table 8.2   Reality Orientation

Reality orientation is a process that helps keep patients with moderate to severe memory loss, confusion, and/or disorientation in touch with the immediate world around them.

- Encompasses all aspects of environment, all hours of the day
- Emphasizes stability in the environment, routine, staff
- Includes frequent, patient reminders of person, time, place
- Uses environmental aids
  - clocks
  - calendars
  - individual color schemes
  - reality boards
- Offers immediate feedback and rewards for success
- Is implemented with respect and patience
  - simple, honest responses to questions
  - calm voice
  - reality-oriented conversations
  - sensitive, caring attitude

Group Classes

- Select four to six patients with similar levels of cognitive function; prepare them individually for the class.
- Assemble group in a quiet, nondistracting environment.
- Put group at ease (offer refreshments, conversation, etc.).
- Identify each patient by name; indicate verbal and nonverbal pleasure at his/her attendance.
- Speak to each patient individually; compliment or otherwise express interest in each as a person.
- Review reality board
  - Today is: Tuesday
  - The date is: March 9
  - The weather is: Cool and windy
  - Our next meal is: Lunch
  - The next holiday is: Easter
- After reviewing the board, ask the group questions related to the board: "What day is it Mr. Smith?", "Mrs. Kent, what kind of weather do we have today?"
- Reward good responses immediately, correct but do not over-react to or dwell on errors.
- Offer a simple activity
  - singing a song
  - picking out pictures of specific items from a magazine
  - exercising
  - planting flowers
- With advanced groups, conduct current events or special topic discussions.
- Limit the group to 15–20 minutes to accommodate limited attention spans.
- It may be useful to assess the mental status of group members at the first session and periodically thereafter; to note any changes that may occur.

- control noise and lighting
- limit traffic flow in environment
- use relaxation techniques (e.g., soft music, warm baths, backrubs, deep breathing, exercise).
- Document specific behaviors (e.g., yelling, slapping, asking same question repeatedly) when giving antipsychotic medications; monitor effect of drug on controlling observable behaviors.

d. Evaluation
- Patient is
  - oriented to person, place, and time.
  - free from injury or secondary complications.

e. Related Possible Nursing Diagnoses
Alteration in health maintenance
Anxiety
Diversional activity deficit
Potential for injury
Powerlessness
Self-care deficit
Sleep pattern disturbance
Social isolation

Selected Health Problems Frequently Associated with the Nursing Diagnosis ALTERATION IN THOUGHT PROCESSES

1. Dementia

a. Definition/Discussion
A general mental deterioration caused by organic or psychologic factors. Some dementias may be reversible, although a majority are not.

This condition is not a normal consequence of growing old although the prevalence does rise with age. Dementia affects less than 3% of persons age 65–74; approximately 6% of persons age 75–49, and over 22% of the population over age 80. Alzheimer's disease is the most common form of irreversible dementia. This condition begins as a mild impairment in cognitive function that can be mistakenly attributed to being busy, eccentric, or absent-minded. As the cognitive impairment continues, the ability to meet basic needs and protect oneself from harm becomes jeopardized. Many times, only the shell of the individual once known remains as aimless wandering, meaningless chatter, decreased emotions, and dependency on others for basic needs become increasingly predominant. This is a devastating disease for the entire family unit. Family members need guidance and support as they confront the disease-related changes of their loved one, assume care-giving responsibilities, and make difficult decisions concerning the welfare of themselves and the Alzheimer's victim. The affected individual needs continued attention to basic needs, protection from hazards, preservation of dignity, and the communication of caring that is important to all human beings.

b. **Etiology**
    – Primary dementias (irreversible)
      • Alzheimer's disease (exact cause unknown, research points to genetic defects, neurotransmitter malfunctions, similarity to pathology of Down's syndrome)
      • presenile (onset before age 60)
      • Senile Dementia of Alzheimer's Type (SDAT) (onset after age 60): responsible for an estimated 50% of all dementia in the elderly
      • multi-infarct dementia (ischemic cerebral lesions): responsible for 15%–20% of elderly dementia
      • alcoholism (Wernicke's encephalopathy)
      • Pick's disease
      • Jakob-Creutzfeld disease
      • Parkinson's disease
      • trauma
      • genetic predisposition
    – Secondary dementias (reversible): responsible for 10% of all dementias
      • metabolic disturbances
      • nutritional deficiency
      • drug intoxication
      • head injuries
      • brain tumors

c. **Clinical Manifestations (primary dementias)**
    – Onset gradual, progressive
    – Decline in intellectual function
      • memory disturbance
      • disorientation
      • decreased conceptual thought
      • impaired abstract thinking
    – Changes in affect
      • reduced frustration level
      • anxiety
      • depression
      • lability
    – Volatile coping reactions, "catastrophic reactions"
      • anger, agitation, sullenness
      • evasiveness, withdrawal

- Decreased attention span
- Preoccupation with self
- Amnesia
- Suspicion, paranoia
- Difficulty in communication, aphasia
- Confabulation
- Delusions (often paranoid)
- Excessive orderliness
- Impaired judgment and decision making
- Poor awareness of surroundings/environmental changes
- Aproxia, impairment of learned movements
- Inability to feed, toilet, or otherwise care for self (later stages)
- Organic brain changes
- *Presenile Alzheimer's*
  • atrophy (detected on brain scan in later stages)
  • widening of sulci
  • narrow convolutions
  • lateral ventricular enlargement
  • reduced white matter
  • cortical neuronal loss
  • senile plaques, neurofibrillary tangles in cortex
- *SDAT*
  • more difficult to diagnose
  • brain changes resemble those of normal aging
- Symmetrical slowing of EEG pattern (not in early stage)

    d. Multidisciplinary Approaches: Symptomatic management

Additional Nursing Care That Can Be Incorporated into the Generic Care Plan

- Provide a safe, structured environment
  • control environmental stimuli
  • place chemicals, medications, and potentially ingestible items out of patient's sight
  • create a defined, limited area for walking/wandering
  • install bells or alarms on doors to signal patient's exit
  • color code or use consistent symbol (e.g., a flower) on patient's room and possessions
- Take patient's anxiety, attention deficit, and intellectual limitations into account when scheduling activities; several short sessions may be preferable to a single long one.
- Monitor intake and output
  • encourage patient to eat; weigh frequently
  • provide easy-to-eat foods and increase caloric intake when restless and wandering
  • regularly remind patient to toilet

- Guide patient in and monitor activities of daily living.
- Give simple, clear directions, one at a time; break tasks into simple steps.
- Orient to reality; do not foster misperception.
- Use consistency in approaches and care.
- Examine patient's body regularly (e.g., during baths) for signs of problems such as skin breakdown, rashes, cuts, bruises, masses.
- Be alert to nonverbal clues of problems (e.g., restlessness, appetite changes, behavior changes, rubbing body part, restricting limb usage, wincing).
- Continuously reassess status and adjust care accordingly.
- Offer support to family members; refer to local Alzheimer's Disease and Related Disorders Association.

2. Delirium

a. Definition/Discussion
A condition marked by defective perception, impaired memory, and a rapid succession of confused and unconnected ideas, often with illusions and hallucinations. A characteristic feature is an altered level of consciousness, ranging from states of stupor to hypervigilance.

Delirium is usually an acute condition, precipitated by exogenous conditions. Once the underlying cause is treated, the person returns to a normal state of functioning.

b. Etiology
- Impairment of cerebral circulation, hypoxia
- Malnutrition, dehydration
- Metabolic imbalance
- Prolonged sleep deprivation
- Congestive heart failure
- Burns
- Reaction to surgery
- Infection
- Alcohol or drug toxicity
- Hyperthermia

c. Clinical Manifestations
- Combativeness, restlessness, agitation
- Insomnia, nightmares
- Tachycardia
- Increased blood pressure
- Apprehension, irritability
- Confusion, disorientation
- Auditory or visual hallucinations
- Illusions, delusions

d. **Multidisciplinary Approaches**
   - Correction of underlying cause
   - Management of symptoms

Additional Nursing Care That Can Be Incorporated into the Generic Care Plan

   - Assess and intervene promptly because condition is reversible and treatment can prevent permanent damage.
   - Use treatment appropriate to cause and note results when treatment is instituted.
   - Provide a quiet environment and adequate lighting to facilitate orientation.
   - Establish a consistent routine.
   - Maintain a stable, moderate room temperature.
   - Prevent injury by patient to self or others.

3. Schizophrenic Disorders

a. **Definition/Discussion**
   Psychotic states characterized by disturbed thinking, withdrawal from reality, regression, and poor interpersonal relationships. There is some thinking that the stresses of old age or a lifetime's accumulation of stresses may intensify pathologic character traits of schizoid personalities. The specialized care needed by the schizophrenic person requires the involvement of a psychiatrist since ineffective management can reduce functional ability and increase the patient's risk of institutionalization.

b. **Etiology:** Unknown, may be the result of
   - Heredity
   - Poor family relationships
   - Traumautic experiences
   - Maladaptive coping
   - Chemical imbalance

c. **Clinical Manifestations**
   - Auditory and visual hallucinations
   - Illogical thinking
   - Incoherence
   - Disorganized thoughts
   - Flat, inappropriate, or silly affect
   - Disorganized or peculiar behavior
   - Poor hygiene, inappropriate dress
   - Social withdrawal and isolation
   - Excited motor activity inconsistent with environmental stimuli

d. Multidisciplinary Approaches
- Medications (antipsychotics)
- Psychotherapy, behavioral therapy

Additional Nursing Care That Can Be Incorporated into the Generic Care Plan

- Maintain a stable environment and routine by limiting patient's contact with unfamiliar people; introduce new staff and explain their function as necessary.
- Help reduce misperceptions by correcting sensory problems (vision or hearing deficits) and avoiding harsh lighting/shadows, unidentified sounds.
- Promote social contact and include patient in reality-oriented activities.
- Prevent complications resulting from peculiar behaviors (e.g., malnutrition, poor hygiene).
- Develop a positive and trusting relationship and provide a safe and secure environment.
- Divert focus from delusional material to reality, and avoid confirming or feeding into delusion.
- Encourage patient to express negative and positive emotions.
- Be familiar with various antipsychotics used to control agitation, delusions, hallucinations and psychotic symptoms (see Table 8.1).
- Be aware that antipsychotic medications are used to help make the patient more receptive to other forms of therapy, not to substitute for other therapies.
- Ensure proper dosage for the older patient
  - one-third to one-half of normal adult dosage is usually prescribed
  - begin with lower dosage and gradually increase to point of maximum benefit/least side effects.
- Observe response to medication carefully as individual responses vary.
- Recognize extrapyramidal side effects (e.g., dyskinesia: involuntary motor movement resembling Parkinson's).
- Assure patient does not consume alcohol or other CNS depressants while taking an antipsychotic.

4. Paranoia

a. Definition/Discussion
A mental disorder characterized by the presence of suspiciousness and delusions. The person often believes others are out to get them (e.g., the FBI, police). A delusion is a fixed belief (false) held with conviction despite evidence to the contrary. When the symptoms are relatively mild, the condition is known as paranoid personality. Paranoic reactions can occur in organic, alcoholic, and other mental illnesses. Paranoid states can be associated with age-related losses that

increase feelings of anxiety, powerlessness, suspiciousness, or with dementia.

b. **Etiology:** Unknown

c. **Clinical Manifestations**
- Suspiciousness, mistrust of others
- Delusions of persecution or grandeur
- Low self-esteem
- High anxiety level
- Hostility toward others
- Self-imposed isolation
- Delusions of having thoughts controlled, messages broadcast to the brain, extraordinary powers

d. **Multidisciplinary Approach:** Psychotherapy

Additional Nursing Care That Can Be Incorporated into the Generic Care Plan

- Establish presence and onset of delusional thoughts; when did unusual behavior become noticeable to others? to the patient?
- Question about specific events surrounding delusional thoughts; they may be a reaction to or exaggeration of a real threat (e.g., fears of personal harm are well founded in residents of high-crime areas).
- Obtain a thorough physical, mental, and social assessment to rule out other possible causes (e.g., organic disorders, trauma).
- Make a special effort to establish rapport.
- Realize that paranoid people desperately need warmth and understanding; do not be put off by patient distrust, accusations.
- Recognize patient's unimpaired intellectual capacity and resentment of being "talked down to."
- Be honest with patient by not supporting delusions, but avoid trying to convince them otherwise; this only reinforces the defense and belief systems.
- Avoid arguing with patient about delusions because the paranoid person can not be rationally talked out of fixed beliefs.
- Prevent patient isolation and focus on reality situations in the environment.
- Monitor impact of paranoia on general health (e.g., nutritional status [fear of poisoning may interfere with food intake]), hygienic practices [patient may refuse to bathe, change clothes because "someone is watching"]).
- Avoid power struggles and arguing with patient because it increases anxiety and hostility.

GENERIC CARE PLAN FOR THE NURSING DIAGNOSIS
IMPAIRED VERBAL COMMUNICATION

1. General Information

Speech and language problems include disorders that interfere with the production, comprehension, or expression of words. Speech and language are not synonymous. *Speech* is the mechanics of producing words; *language* is the comprehension and expression of ideas. People can have speech problems, language problems, or a combination of both. Effective nursing care depends upon knowing the specific cause of the speech/language problem. Early rehabilitative measures can decrease psychologic trauma and promote normal function and independence.

a. Etiology
  – Motor disorders that interfere with word formation
  – Neurologic disturbances that limit comprehension, expression
  – Mental problems that alter word organization, interpretation
  – Hearing deficits that decrease or distort received word
  – Ethnic/cultural identity that causes linguistic differences between patient and nurse

b. Clinical Manifestations
  – Aphasia: loss of language function, usually due to problems within the central nervous system; can be *expressive*, where there is an inability to communicate thoughts verbally or in writing due to a motor problem; *receptive*, with an inability to comprehend language due to sensory problem; or *mixed*, a combination of expressive and receptive
  – Dysphasia: impaired use of words; can be *receptive*, in which patient can not understand words; or *expressive*, in which patient can not organize words correctly or use right name for a person or object
  – Dysarthria: problem with articulation due to poor motor control of the lips, tongue, and/or pharynx; will use correct word but have difficulty pronouncing it
  – Paraphasia: a mild form of aphasia in which one word is substituted for another (e.g., clock for watch)

c. Multidisciplinary Approach: Speech therapy

2. Nursing Process

a. Assessment
  – Lip, tongue motion
  – Soft palate symmetry

- Vocal cord movement
- Gag reflex swallowing
- Respiration
- Articulation (speed and quality)
- Hearing
- Simple tests of language difficulty
  - show five everyday objects and ask the name of each (e.g., pen, paperclip, cup, book, comb)
  - put the objects aside then have the patient point to each as you name it
  - ask the patient to repeat several simple sentences after you
  - state an expression or truism and ask the patient to explain its meaning (e.g., "People in glass houses shouldn't throw stones . . . "; "A bird in hand is worth two in the bush.")
  - have patient repeat "ma, ma, ma" (tests motor control of lips); use "la, la, la" (tests tongue), "ga, ga, ga" (tests pharynx); note distortions and slurring.

b. Goal
Patient will be able to communicate needs and comprehend what is being said.

c. Interventions
- Determine the patient's actual deficits and capabilities.
- Describe the speech or language impairment to the patient (if possible), the family, and all care givers.
- Treat the patient like an intelligent adult; realize that an inability to form words does not necessitate talking as if to a child or shouting.
- Keep the patient oriented by describing current events, introducing care givers, and explaining activities.
- Maximize existing strengths by using visual cues and assistive devices such as flash cards and communication boards containing common words for the patient to point to; pen and paper; synthesizers and other assistive devices as recommended by the therapist.
- Be patient and accepting of the patient's impairment; allow patient time to process words.
- Promote socialization and diversion; encourage family to visit, talk to patient during care activities.
- Refer speech and language problems to a speech pathologist for thorough examination.

d. Evaluation
- Patient
  - participates in activities of daily living to maximum degree possible.
  - communicates effectively.

e. **Possible Related Nursing Diagnoses**
Anxiety
Disturbance in self-concept
Fear
Impaired social interaction
Potential for injury
Potential social isolation
Sensory-perceptual alteration

GENERIC CARE PLAN FOR THE NURSING DIAGNOSIS
SENSORY-PERCEPTUAL ALTERATION

1. General Information

Sensory-perceptual alterations exist when the usual and accustomed sensory stimuli are not experienced or recognized accurately. The individual experiences a change in the amount, pattern, or interpretation of incoming stimuli as a result of physiologic, sensory, motor, or environmental disruptions. The age-related declines in sensory organ function predispose the elderly to major impairments in recognizing and interpreting incoming sensory stimuli. Hearing loss is the reduced ability of sounds to be transmitted and/or perceived by the ear. Presbycusis is a sensorineural hearing loss experienced with age and is a common problem of the elderly. With this type of loss there is a loss of high-frequency sounds followed by middle- and low-frequency sound losses as the hearing deficit progresses. Conductive hearing losses can accompany sensorineural losses, further distorting incoming sounds.

a. **Etiology**
   – Age-related changes to sensory organs (e.g., presbycusis)
   – Neurologic disease
     • cerebrovascular accident
     • neuropathies
   – Musculoskeletal problems
     • paralysis
   – Medications
     • sedatives
     • tranquilizers
     • ototoxic drugs: salicylates, streptomycin, kanamycin
   – Environmental factors
     • change in environment
     • high or multiple noise stimuli
     • poor lighting
   – Recurrent ear, eye, or upper respiratory infections
   – Ear wax accumulation

– Physical or social isolation
– Trauma

b. Clinical Manifestations
– Vision, hearing deficits
– Inappropriate responses or behaviors
– Disorientation, confusion
– Anxiety, fear
– Suspiciousness
– Visual or auditory hallucinations
– Restlessness, sleep disturbances
– Inattention
– Inappropriate response
– Unusually loud speech
– Requests to have words repeated
– Cocking head in the direction of the "good" ear
– Paranoia (believe others are talking about them or whispering behind their backs)

c. Multidisciplinary Approaches
– Evaluate medication and effects
– Surgery to correct condition
– Corrective/assistive devices (eyeglasses, hearing aids)

2. Nursing Process

a. Assessment
– History of symptoms patient is experiencing
  • onset
  • precipitating factors
  • frequency
  • pattern
  • how relieved or improved on
– Impact on patient's total well-being and life-style
– Visual ability
  • ensure that a thorough ophthalmologic exam has been done
  • determine if the patient can read large print, differentiate items on a food tray, count fingers held in front of him or her, recognize faces, notice only shadows, see items in a restricted visual field, etc.
  • read Snellen chart, newsprint (with and without eyeglasses), visual fields (see Table 8.3)
– Hearing
  • inspect ear with otoscope; note swelling, redness, drainage, cerumen, foreign material
  • hear normal conversation, watch ticking, whisper, consonants
  • *Weber test*: A vibrating tuning fork is placed on the forehead. If

sensorineural loss is present, patient will hear tone in unimpaired ear; if a conductive loss is present, will hear tone better in impaired ear. With equal bilateral deafness or normal hearing, tones will be heard equally in both ears.
  • *Rinne test*: A vibrating tuning fork is placed on the mastoid process (bony prominence behind ear) then removed and held alongside the ear. If a conductive loss is present, the tone will be heard louder on the mastoid process; if a sensorineural loss is present or hearing is normal, tone will be louder alongside the ear; if a combined conductive and sensorineural loss is present, the tone will be heard equally at both locations.
  – Ability to differentiate different tactile stimuli (cold-hot, sharp-dull)
  – Ability to identify various scents (vinegar, coffee, perfume)
  – Ability to taste different substances (lemon, salt, sugar)
  – Explore environment for contributory factors

b. **Goal**
Patient will receive and interpret adequate sensory stimuli to protect self from hazards and accurately perceive reality of environment.

c. **Interventions**
  – Remove or minimize cause
    • control noise
    • adjust lighting
    • encourage use of eyeglasses, hearing aids
    • correct sensory deprivation or overload
    • promote physical health (stabilization of vital signs, restore fluid and electrolyte imbalance)
    • consult with physician regarding medication change

Table 8.3   Assessing Visual Fields

This test provides a gross estimation of visual field and can be helpful in understanding adjustments that may have to be made in care. An ophthalmologist can test visual field with a target screen to obtain the most accurate evaluation.

1. Seat patient comfortably.
2. Position yourself approximately 3 feet away facing the patient at eye level.
3. Point your index finger and extend your arm so that it is out of your visual field.
4. Ask the patient to stare into your eyes as you stare into the patient's.
5. As you and the patient continue to stare, slowly bring your finger into the visual field.
6. Ask the patient to inform you when s/he first can see your finger.
7. Note when patient sees finger compared to when you do.
8. Repeat at various points along a 360° area of the visual field.
9. Record deficits in patient's chart so that care givers can plan accordingly. (Sample entry: Extremely limited peripheral vision in left field. Intervention: Position bed so that right side faces door; keep bedside stand on right side.)

- Provide adequate sensory stimulation
  - determine appropriate and desired level for individual
  - keep patient oriented with use of clocks, calendars, windows to see daylight and darkness
  - use different fabrics, colors, fragrances in environment
  - flavor foods (use artificial sweeteners and salt substitutes if restrictions are needed)
  - offer music, art therapy.
- Explain actions, clarify misconceptions.
- Protect patient from injury
  - limit temperature of hot water
  - color-code faucet handles
  - keep stairways well lighted
  - label liquids and other substances well, do not store noningestible substances near ingestible ones
  - elicit aid from roommate or family member to observe for hazards.
- *Hearing deficits*
  - remove cerumen if present; soften wax with cerumenolytic agent then irrigate with body temperature water under low pressure; avoid using cotton-tipped applicators since they can push cerumen further into canal and cause it to impact.
  - communicate in a manner that maximizes the patient's strengths
    * face directly, attract patient's attention before beginning to speak
    * speak slowly and distinctly
    * use a loud but low-pitched voice: raising the voice in a yelling manner will raise a high-frequency sound even higher and cause the patient to understand less of what is spoken
    * supplement words with exaggerated facial movements and body language
    * give the patient the opportunity to ask for clarification or repetition.
  - promote optimum communication at night or in darkened room
    * use a night light
    * have ample light shining on you so that the patient can easily detect your presence and not be startled
    * touch the patient to gain attention
    * use a flashlight to light your face, facilitate lip reading
    * avoid interrupting other persons who may be sleeping in the same room by using a stethoscope to amplify speech; place the earpieces in the patient's ear and talk into the bell/diaphragm portion; explain procedure to the patient beforehand.
  - write down instructions and important information to ensure patient understanding.
  - consult with an occupational therapist about recommendations for assistive devices (e.g., speaking tube, telephone with special amplifier, light signals rather than sound alarms).
  - ensure that patient is not avoided or socially isolated.

- counsel patient about hearing aid use
  * hearing aids do not benefit persons with sensorineural loss
  * even with conductive losses, hearing aids can be a problem and difficult to adjust to because all environmental sounds are amplified also.
- instruct patient on proper use and care of hearing aid (see Table 8.4).
- *Vision deficits*
  - always identify yourself when approaching the patient.
  - help strangers recognize patient's visual problems by providing a white cane or placing a sign on the bedroom door.
  - place patient's belongings and items on food tray in same location at all times to facilitate independent functioning.
  - make a special effort to keep the patient oriented
    * read newspapers and books to patient (read mail only after asking if he or she wishes for you to do so)

Table 8.4 Hearing Aids

Components

Microphone: converts sounds into electric energy
Amplifier: increases energy
Receiver: converts energy back into sound waves
Volume control
On/off switch

Styles

Behind the ear: limited amplification
In the ear: entire unit worn in the ear; limited amplification
Eyeglass attached: unit built in the frame of the eyeglass; limited amplification
Body aided: amplifier housed in a case worn on body; offers most amplification of all

Nursing Care

−Encourage patient to obtain hearing aid from a reputable dealer after a full audiometric examination has been done.
−Ensure that batteries are functioning before the aid is applied; it is recommended that batteries be changed weekly.
−Identify common hearing aid problems
  • whistling sound: bad connection between earpiece and amplifier; excessively high volume
  • insufficient amplification: volume set too low; weak or dead battery; blockage from cerumen; disconnected tubing or wiring
  • periodic loss of amplification: loose connection; poor battery contact; dirt in switch; cracked case
−Clean device weekly to remove cerumen and dirt
  • rotate a pipe cleaner in the opening of the earmold to remove material
  • wash earmold in warm soapy water
  • thoroughly dry
  • do not use alcohol or alcohol-based substances for cleaning
−Turn off when not in use.
−Keep away from excessive heat or cold.
−Recognize that adjustment to a hearing aid is difficult and may take time. Reassure the patient that this is not unusual.

* describe colors and layout of surroundings
* have a radio available; use clocks that chime.
• assist the patient with mobility and transfers
    * have patient hold your arm above elbow rather than you holding patient, and walk naturally
    * warn patient when approaching stairs or curbs; describe depth and number
    * when seating patient describe where seat is; place patient's hand on back of seat for orientation.
• Ensure safety of environment
    * keep doors completely open or closed
    * remove cords, furniture, buckets, and other obstacles from patient's path
    * keep bed cranks in and slippers out of the way.
• explore with occupational therapist or local service agencies the use of assistive devices (e.g., large print or braille books, games and telephone dials, talking books); the American Foundation for the Blind (15 West 15 Street, New York, NY 10011) can supply a catalog with hundreds of useful items.
• support patient's independence and involvement in social and life activities.

d. Evaluation
Patient
– Is free from secondary problems resulting from sensory-perceptual alterations.
– Receives satisfactory level of sensory input to maintain safety and orientation, and to obtain pleasure from surroundings.

e. Possible Related Nursing Diagnoses
Anxiety
Disturbance in self-concept
Impaired social interaction
Impaired verbal communication
Potential for injury
Potential social isolation

Selected Health Problems Frequently Associated with the Nursing Diagnosis SENSORY-PERCEPTUAL ALTERATION

1. Cataract

a. Definition
A slowly developing opacity of the lens or its capsule. Most elderly

persons have some degree of cataract formation, which can cause visual impairments ranging from a sensitivity to glare to blindness.

b. **Etiology**
    – Aging process (senile cataract)
    – Congenital
    – Eye trauma or disease

c. **Clinical Manifestations**
    – Gray or white opacity over pupil
    – Blurred vision
    – Increased sensitivity to glare
    – Progressive loss of vision
    – Painless

d. **Multidisciplinary Approaches**
    – Surgical removal of cataracts
      • extracapsular extraction: the simplest procedure, which removes the lens leaving the posterior capsule in place
      • intracapsular extraction: the procedure most commonly performed for the elderly, which removes both lens and capsule.

Additional Nursing Care That Can Be Incorporated into the Generic Care Plan

– Inspect eye for gray or white opacity.
– Review history for onset and progression of visual problems, diseases present, and trauma to eye.
– Arrange for ophthalmalogic examination.
– Reduce glare with sunglasses and translucent coverings on windows to filter sunlight; use soft lights to diffuse lighting.
– Protect unaffected eye.
– Place objects within visual field.
– Monitor eye health by watching the progress of cataract and the status of unaffected eye.
– Prepare patient for operation by
  • explaining operative procedure and postoperative routines
  • orienting patient to the position of items in the room
  • emphasizing the importance of limiting intraocular pressure (e.g., avoid coughing, sneezing, bending)
  • applying mydriatics (eye drops to dilate the eye) and antibiotic ophthalmic ointments as prescribed.
– Give postoperative care
  • focus on patient's comfort
  • observe for signs of complications (sudden eye pain, changes in vital signs)
  • consult physician about proper care of soft contact or permanent intraocular implant lenses
  • encourage independence as soon as possible.

2. Glaucoma

a. Definition
An increase of pressure within the eyeball due to increased production and/or decreased outflow of aqueous humor. It is the second leading cause of blindness in the elderly.

b. Etiology
– Iritis
– Allergy
– Endocrine imbalance
– Familial tendency

c. Clinical Manifestations
– Chronic glaucoma (most common type)
  • eyes feel tired
  • gradually increasing impairment of peripheral vision
  • halo around lights
  • headaches (particularly in the morning)
– Acute glaucoma
  • severe eye pain
  • nausea, vomiting
  • halo around lights
  • dilated pupils
  • blurred vision that can progress rapidly to blindness if untreated

d. Multidisciplinary Approaches
– Medications
  • parasympathomimetics (miotics)
  • sympathomimetics
  • carbonic anhydrase inhibitors
  • hyperosmotic agents
– Surgery
  • corneoscleral trephine
  • iridencleisis
  • sclerectomy
  • cyclocryotherapy

Additional Nursing Care That Can Be Incorporated into the Generic Care Plan

– Obtain history of symptoms and evaluate visual field (see Table 8.3).
– Arrange for ophthalmologic examination with tonometry, a simple test for measuring intraocular pressure.
– Encourage regular glaucoma screening in *all* elderly patients (glau-

coma is second only to cataracts in frequency among older persons with eye disease).

- Teach the patient to avoid situations that increase intraocular pressures
  - coughing, sneezing, aggressive nose blowing
  - strenuous exercise
  - constipation, straining during defecation
  - emotional stress
- Assess the extent of the visual defects and assist patient with activities of daily living as needed.
- Counsel patient to use eyes in moderation and prevent overuse or strain.
- Protect patient from accidental administration of drugs (e.g., stimulants, blood pressure elevators).
- Advise patient to inform care givers of presence of glaucoma when new medications are prescribed or administered.
- Warn patient against self-prescription with over-the-counter medications, particularly cold and allergy remedies and diet aids (they increase intraocular pressure).
- It may be useful for patient to wear a bracelet or other identifying tag that will inform others of the problem if the patient cannot.
- Ensure regular evaluation by an ophthalmologist to monitor intraocular pressure and adjust treatment if necessary.

GENERIC CARE PLAN FOR THE NURSING DIAGNOSIS
ALTERATION IN COMFORT: PAIN

1. General Information

Pain is a state in which the individual experiences an uncomfortable sensation in response to a noxious stimulus. *Acute* pain is time limited, and can be relieved (e.g., toothache, postoperative myocardial infarction). *Chronic* pain has no predictable time limitations and only limited relief by conventional analgesics (e.g., arthritis, shingles, phantom limb, migraine, terminal cancer). In the elderly, pain often presents itself in an altered manner, being referred to another area from its origin (e.g., gallbladder disorders can cause pain in the shoulder area) or bearing no relationship to the severity of the problem (e.g., a myocardial infarction may cause only a fluttering sensation in the chest).

a. Etiology
- Improper positioning, restrictive clothing
- Noise level, uncomfortable temperature
- Actual or potential tissue damage
- Trauma, disease process

b. Clinical Manifestations
- Complaining of pain, discomfort, nausea
- Stabbing, aching, throbbing sensations
- Diaphoresis, pallor
- Requests for pain medication
- Increased vital signs
- Crying, grimacing
- Restless, irritable
- Altered mood or behavior (confusion, depression, anxiety, irritability)

c. Multidisciplinary Approaches
- Analgesics (see Table 8.5)
- Surgical intervention
- Chemical rhizotomy
- Transcutaneous electrical nerve stimulation (TENS)

2. Nursing Process

a. Assessment
- Individual pain pattern, type of pain, pain threshold
- Precipitating factors and all sources of discomfort
- Frequency, duration, and intensity of pain
- Alleviating factors
- Ethnic, religious, or sexual influences on the expression of pain
- Impact on daily life (e.g., food intake, mobility, social contact)

b. Goals
Patient
- will experience increased comfort with the implementation of nonpharmaceutical methods of pain control.
- will experience pain relief by the proper administration of analgesics.

c. Interventions
- Assure maximum comfort by good positioning, physical support, and clean, wrinkle-free linens.
- Control environmental stimuli; alter the room temperature, provide warm or cool clothing as indicated, reduce noise level and external stimuli if it is contributing to the pain perception.
- Gently touch patient (e.g., rub brow, massage, backrub, hold hand) to promote relaxation and comfort; utilize relaxation techniques, guided imagery, biofeedback, hypnosis.
- Allow patient to express feelings of anger, powerlessness, anxiety.
- Be alert to newly developed symptoms or multiple complaints (e.g., knee and ankle pain may be attributed to previously diagnosed arthritis, but really arise from new vascular problem).
- Review patient's own pain-relief regimen to facilitate treatment by

Table 8.5   Analgesics

Examples	Common Side Effects	Nursing Implications
Non-narcotics		
Acetaminophen Aspirin	Irritating to gastric mucosa Prolonged bleeding time, GI bleeding (aspirin) Salicylate toxicity: tinnitus, hearing loss, dizziness, vomiting, burning in mouth, throat, sweating, fever, confusion, convulsions, coma	Be alert to signs of infection (can mask associated fever). Give with food or milk to reduce risk of gastric bleeding/irritation; follow with a full glass of water; do not give aspirin with fruit juice. Observe for increased bleeding tendency (bruising, bleeding gums). Can alter test readings for glycosuria.
Narcotics		
Codeine Morphine Meperidine	Drowsiness, dizziness Skin rash, itching Nausea, vomiting Hypotension, bradycardia Constipation Dependence Exaggeration of existing mental impairment Severe depressant reaction in the elderly Interference with urination	Protect from accidents. Reduce dosage if recommended.
Brompton's mixture (combination of methadone, ethyl alcohol, cocaine, hydrochloride syrup)		Used primarily in terminal illness Administered orally (every four hours); effective within 30 minutes

Interactions

Non-narcotics

- Increase effect of cortisonelike drugs, oral anticoagulants, oral antidiabetics, penicillins, furosemide, para-aminosalicylic acid (PAS) (greater risk of aspirin toxicity).
- Decrease effect of probenecid, spironolactone, sulfinpyrazone.
- Effects increased by large doses of vitamin C.
- Effects decreased by antacids, phenobarbital, propranolol, reserpine.

Narcotics

- Increase effect of antidepressants, other analgesics, sedatives, tranquilizers.
- Effects increased by antidepressants, phenothiazines, nitrates (meperidine).
- Effects decreased by eye drops prescribed for glaucoma (meperidine).

identifying successful practices and reveal additional problems (e.g., inappropriate medication use, dangerous or ineffective "fad" cures).
- Minimize impact of pain on total health by preserving energy, providing adequate nutrition, encouraging eating and activity.
- Perform range-of-motion exercises if mobility is reduced.
- Maintain independence, normality, and individuality.
- Assess need for medication and evaluate effectiveness (see Table 8.5)
  - begin with weakest form of analgesics; increase gradually
  - remember that non-narcotics will be less sedating; will have fewer, less severe side effects; and are nonaddictive
  - administer analgesia regularly to maintain constant blood levels, maximize relief
  - administer narcotic analgesics with caution in the elderly; there can be serious side effects, psychologic and physiologic dependency
  - give non-narcotic analgesics with narcotics to reduce required narcotic dosage
  - monitor vital signs carefully (particularly respiration) in all persons receiving narcotics.

d. **Evaluation**
   - Patient
     - verbalizes comfort, absence or decrease of pain.
     - experiences less pain.
     - participates in activities of daily living to maximum degree possible.

e. **Possible Related Nursing Diagnoses**
   Activity intolerance
   Alteration in nutrition
   Anxiety
   Impaired social interaction
   Powerlessness
   Self-care deficit
   Sleep pattern disturbance

GENERIC CARE PLAN FOR THE NURSING DIAGNOSIS
KNOWLEDGE DEFICIT

1. General Information

Knowledge deficit is a state in which the individual experiences a deficiency in cognitive knowledge or psychomotor skills that alters or may alter health maintenance.

a. **Etiology**
    – Sensory deficit
       • visual impairment
       • poor hearing
    – Ineffective coping
       • denial
       • anxiety
    – Alzheimer's disease
    – New illness or treatment
    – Cultural practices, language differences
    – Impaired learning ability, cognitive deficit
    – Ineffective teaching

b. **Clinical Manifestations**
    – Expresses lack of knowledge or inaccurate knowledge
    – Noncompliance with health practices or medical treatment
    – Appears to be anxious or depressed, resulting from misinformation or lack of information

c. **Multidisciplinary Approaches**
    – Referral to necessary experts (e.g., dieticians, enterostomal therapists)
    – Outside resources (e.g., American Cancer Society)
    – Social Worker

2. Nursing Process

a. **Assessment**
    – Clarify with the patient what is to be taught (e.g., what constitutes a good diet or why it is important that dietary practices be changed)
    – Learning ability
       • intellectual capacity (memory, attention span, communication skills, problem-solving capability)
       • learning and skills (literacy, counting, educational achievements, knowledge base)
       • psychomotor skills (motor dexterity, balance, equilibrium, sensation, mobility)
       • emotional capacity (acceptance of illness or physical limitations, control, self-image, motivation)
       • physical capacity (energy level, vision, hearing, speech, general health)
    – Current knowledge level
       • previous experience
       • independent learning
       • beliefs

b. **Goals**

Patient
- will participate in the learning process.
- will learn necessary procedures and initiate necessary life-style changes.

c. **Interventions**
- Prepare the patient for the education experience by explaining the purpose of the instruction.
- Try to arrange a specific time in advance so that patients can prepare themselves, invite family members, avoid scheduling other activities, etc.
- Provide an environment conducive to learning that is quiet, clean, private, relaxing, and odor free.
- Give instruction time to the patient exclusively with no interruptions.
- Select a teaching method appropriate to patient's abilities and needs
  - a highly educated patient may benefit from reading materials and follow-up discussion
  - an illiterate may require a diagrammed flipchart presentation followed by an audio tape left at bedside for repeated review
  - literature may be sufficient to reach a diabetic diet, but people require "hands-on" practice with needle and syringe for insulin administration.
- Use a variety of methods to present the content: lecture, flipcharts, diagrams, pamphlets, books, demonstrations, audiovisual media, group sessions, discussions with other patients.
- Determine priorities (e.g., of the many different facts taught to newly diagnosed diabetics, how to administer insulin and eat properly are of more immediate concern than recognizing possible complications).
- Close with a summary of content and an opportunity for the patient to ask questions.
- Leave written material describing the content presented for the patient's and family's later review; write a summary in the style and level of language the patient understands.
- Evaluate the effectiveness of the education
  - obtain feedback from patient and family
  - observe the patient for use of new knowledge
  - ask questions informally, at a later time, to confirm understanding.
- Document what was taught, when, who was involved and program effectiveness for the benefit of other team members.
- Know that local, public, and college libraries, health departments, federal information services, professional organizations, and special interest groups can provide excellent supplementary and educational materials.

d. Evaluation
  − Patient
    • verbalizes accurate knowledge pertaining to condition and related care.
    • demonstrates behaviors consistent with desired practices.
    • complies with treatment plan.

e. Possible Related Nursing Diagnoses
  Alteration in health maintenance
  Noncompliance
  Potential for injury
  Anxiety
  Powerlessness

References

American College of Physicians Report (1983). Toward an effective treatment of Alzheimer's disease. *Annals of Internal Medicine, 98*(251).

Anderson, S., & Bauwens, E. (1981). *Chronic health problems: Concepts and applications.* St. Louis: Mosby.

Brink, T. (1979). *Geriatric psychotherapy.* New York: Human Sciences Press.

Butler, R., & Lewis, M. (1982). *Aging and mental health. Positive psychosocial and biomedical approaches* (3rd ed.). St. Louis: Mosby.

Clites, J. (1984). Maximizing memory retention in the aged. *Journal of Gerontological Nursing, 10*(8), 34−35, 38−39.

Dietsche, L., & Pollman, J. (1983). Alzheimer's disease: Advances in clinical nursing. *Journal of Gerontological Nursing, 8*(2), 33−36.

Eifrig, D., & Simons, K. (1983). An overview of common geriatric ophthalmologic disorders. *Geriatrics, 38*(4), 55−79.

Fisher, M. (1984). Peripheral neuropathies: A common complaint in older patients. *Geriatrics, 39*(2), 115−129.

Gilmore, R. (1984). Movement disorders in the aged. *Geriatrics, 39*(6), 65−76.

Hart, G. (1983). Strokes causing left versus right hemiplegia: Different effects and nursing implications. *Geriatric Nursing, 4*(1), 39−43.

Hiatt, R. (1983). Blindness: The physician's role in prevention. *Geriatrics, 38*(12), 97−99.

Kasper, R. (1983). Eye problems of the aged. In W. Reichel (Ed.), *Clinical aspects of aging* (2nd ed.). Baltimore: Williams & Wilkins.

Katzman, R. (Ed.). (1983). *Biological aspects of Alzheimer's disease.* Cold Spring Harbor: Cold Springs Harbor Laboratory.

Kohut, S., Kohut, J., & Fleishman, J. (1983). *Reality orientation for the elderly* (2nd ed.). Oradell, NJ: Medical Economics Books.

Levy, R., & Post, F. (Eds.). (1982). *The psychiatry of late life.* Boston: Blackwell.

Mace, N. (1984). Facets of dementia. *Journal of Gerontological Nursing, 10*(38).

Nemos, M. (1985). Functional assessment of the patient with Alzheimer's disease. *Geriatric Nursing, 6*(3), 139−142.

Price, L., & Snider, R. (1983). The geriatric patient: Ear, nose and throat problems. In W. Reichel (Ed.), *Clinical aspects of aging* (2nd ed.). Baltimore: Williams & Wilkins.

Rabins, P., & Folstein, M. (1983). The demented patient: Evaluation and care. *Geriatrics, 38*(8), 99−106.

Robbins, S. (1978). Stroke in the geriatric patient. In W. Reichel (Ed.), *The geriatric patient.* New York: HP Publishing.

Schafter, S. (1985). Modifying the environment of patients with Alzheimer's disease. *Geriatric Nursing, 6*(3), 157–159.

Schneider, E. (1985). Alzheimer's disease: Research highlights. *Geriatric Nursing, 6*(3), 136–138.

Strub, R., & Black, F. (1981). *Organic brain syndrome: An introduction to neurobehavioral disorders.* Philadelphia: Davis.

Weinstock, F. (1983). Managing geriatric vision problems: Where to get help. *Geriatrics, 38*(5), 96–102.

Weinstock, F. (1983). When to refer to an ophthalmologist. *Geriatrics, 38*(11), 117–124.

Wolanin, M., & Phillips, L. (1981). *Confusion: Prevention and care.* St. Louis: Mosby.

CHAPTER 9

SELF-PERCEPTION/ COPING-STRESS TOLERANCE
FUNCTIONAL HEALTH PATTERN

Today's older population has confronted challenges and obstacles unknown to younger generations, such as world wars, the Great Depression, and epidemics. They also have faced a profoundly rapid rate of change that has required adaptation to new technologies, behaviors, and ways of thinking. The fact that most elderly have survived and adjusted to these situations is a credit to their strength and coping capacity. However, old age brings a new set of stresses—retirement, deaths, illness, role changes—at a time when physical and emotional reserves are declining. Effective management of these stresses is crucial to prevent additional problems.

Under normal circumstances people usually have a fairly realistic image of themselves. They understand their significance, capabilities, and limitations. However, under stress and other circumstances, individuals may lose their perspective and develop altered perceptions of themselves and their world.

Distortions in perception occur when one's anxiety escalates from a moderate to a severe level. Narrowed perception and an inability to take in new information is a common manifestation of high anxiety. The individual has difficulty hearing, learning or remembering information.

Many of the realities of old age make the elderly vulnerable to self-perception problems. Older adults suffer numerous losses, have less ability to protect themselves and fewer resources, and are confronted with many subtle messages of their undesirability in a youth-oriented society. Depression

221

often creates negative and distorted perceptions about self-worth, abilities to succeed, and meaningfulness in life. It is no wonder many begin to feel vulnerable and view themselves negatively.

Coping with chronic illness is a predicament that many elderly people deal with on an ongoing basis. Most older persons suffer from at least one chronic disease and often, several chronic diseases are managed simultaneously. Life-style and normal activities may need to be altered to meet care requirements and limitations. Self-concept and role identity may be threatened. Financial burdens may ensue from the cost of illness management and reduced employment. The shift in roles and responsibilities increase the patient's dependency on other family members. There are constraints on social activity if the patient function is limited. Overwhelmed by physical, emotional, and financial burdens, physical and emotional health of family members is slowly eroded.

The awareness of a need to adapt to a new life-style and awareness of lifelong, perhaps progressive, illness often leads to depression. Periodic episodes are common and are characterized by lack of interest in self-care, withdrawal, or suicidal comments or actions. The inability to face the profound reality of chronic disease can cause the patient to deny the existence of the disease. Characterized by such comments as "No one told me my diabetes wouldn't go away" and unrealistic behaviors (e.g., a terminally ill person planning a world cruise for the following year). Denial may occur after the patient has seemed to accept the illness.

Some people react with manipulation to assure needs are fulfilled. They need to seek attention or exercise control during times of loss. Manipulation is frequently characterized by increased dependency, involving a series of requests and instilling guilt in others. Hostility is an expression of the bitterness at being a victim of a serious illness. Anger is often displaced on close relations or companion (e.g., family members or care givers). Regression occurs when the illness becomes too overwhelming to manage psychologically or physically. Patients relinquish responsibility for self-care or retreat to a lesser level of functioning.

GENERIC CARE PLAN FOR THE NURSING DIAGNOSIS
DISTURBANCE IN SELF-CONCEPT

1. General Information

Disturbance in self-concept is the state in which the individual experiences, or is at risk of experiencing, negative feelings about him/herself. It may be triggered by a change in body image, self-esteem, role performance, or personal identity. The physical, emotional, and social losses experienced with age play a significant role in altering the elderly's self-concept.

a. **Etiology**
   - Change or loss of role (retirement, widowhood)
   - Changes in body appearance or function
   - Dependency

b. **Clinical Manifestations**
   - Anger
   - Withdrawal
   - Grief, depression
   - Denial of problem
   - Self-destructive actions
   - New or increased dependency
   - Preoccupation with change or loss
   - Not taking responsibility for self-care

c. **Multidisciplinary Approaches**
   - Corrective surgery, prosthetic devices
   - Psychotherapy

2. Nursing Process

a. **Assessment**
   - Underlying cause
   - Impact of change on activities, roles, relationships, self-esteem
   - Assistive devices or efforts that have been tried and their success
   - Disturbed body image, behavioral disorganization, distortions, level of anxiety
   - Signs of grieving, withdrawn behavior and use of denial

b. **Goal**
   Patient will be able to regain a positive image of self and engage in normal activities.

c. **Interventions**
   - Assist in regaining maximum function and acceptable appearance (e.g., support, rehabilitative program, use of prosthetic devices).
   - Encourage social interactions with significant others.
   - Discuss new roles with patient and encourage a process of self-discovery in establishing an altered life-style.
   - Recognize accomplishments, give sincere praise.
   - Provide opportunities for feelings to be expressed.
   - Discuss the meaning the loss or change has for the patient.
   - Set limits on maladaptive behaviors and identify positive behaviors that will develop adaptive coping.
   - Encourage patient to make decisions and follow through on plans.
   - Refer to support groups, counseling as necessary.

- Allow time for the grieving process and inform patient of the need to grieve for loss (see Grief).
- Encourage patient to reminisce about the past in order to gain a perspective on life (see Table 9.1).
- Provide time and encouragement for patients to discuss their lives.
- Explore patients' expressed disappointments and frustrations with their lives or selves (e.g., rather than respond to the patient's remark that he feels he made a mess of his life with the statement "No you didn't . . . now don't talk like that," use reflection and open-ended questions to help the patient express and explore the issues).
- Help patients to learn new skills and find new roles.
- Assist patients to find pleasure and meaning in life, regardless of level of function or desirability (e.g., doing for others, maintaining religious practices, developing a family history book or other legacy for future generations).

d. **Evaluation**
- Patient
  • develops new roles and functions to replace lost ones.
  • accepts altered appearance, function, or roles.

e. **Possible Related Nursing Diagnoses**
Alteration in family processes
Alteration in parenting
Anxiety
Impaired physical mobility
Ineffective individual coping
Powerlessness
Sensory-perceptual alteration
Sexual dysfunction

Selected Health Problems Frequently Associated with the Nursing Diagnosis DISTURBANCE IN SELF-CONCEPT

1. Depression

a. **Definition/Discussion**
A feeling of extreme sadness, self-depreciation, and lack of interest in activities of daily living. It is different from grief, which has realistic and proportionate feelings related to a real loss. Depression is thought to affect some 3% of the general population and is more prevalent among the elderly. Some degree of depression exists in an estimated

Table 9.1   Reminiscence

Reminiscence is a therapeutic review of one's past life to

-resolve current conflicts
-illuminate the individual's past
-organize and understand significance of past events
-cope with the present and future
-maximize use of long-term memory when short-term memory is poor
-offer a comfortable mechanism for expressing self more comfortably
-maintain identity and self-esteem

Use reminiscence to assess

-individual accomplishments, needs
-self-esteem
-cognitive function
-emotional stability
-unresolved conflicts
-coping ability
-expectations for the future

Group Process

Use questions to initiate and guide reminiscence. Strategies could include

-Listening actively and with interest to discussions of patients' lives.
-Helping patients compile poems, oral histories, or scrapbooks of their lives.
-Asking patients to share information about their past. Questions could include "What was it like to leave Europe and come to America?" "How did you celebrate holidays as a child?" "What were your parents and grandparents like?" "Did you have any pets when you were young?" "How did you spend your time as a teenager?" "What was the factory like when you started working there?"
-Playing old songs and showing old photos, newspapers or magazines, and asking what was happening in the patient's life at that time.
-Structuring intergenerational activities in which the old can share their past with the young.
-Respecting patients' privacy so that periods of silent reminiscing are not disturbed.
-Asking patients to talk about a specific event or time (e.g., "Tell me how it was to be a girl in Germany." "What was your first job like?" "What was the city like when you were a teenager?").
-Using questions to help patients explore emotional responses to past events (e.g., "How did you feel when your town was invaded during the war?" "How difficult was it for you as a young widow?" "Were you disappointed at having to quit school?").
-Gently redirecting the conversation if patients' responses are repetitious or aimless (e.g., "you mentioned that before . . . did that event have a special meaning for you?" "Let's get back to how you began your career." "How do you feel about the problems you describe between yourself and your family?").
-Listening to patients' responses; this is the most important nursing function in reminiscence.
-Informing patients of time constraints and enforcing them; if appropriate, ask patients to summarize or identify the lesson/theme of the conversation.

50%–80% of all institutionalized persons. Depression can also occur early in dementia as the patient becomes aware of intellectual decline.

b. **Etiology**
   – Reduced levels of norepinephrine, serotinin or their metabolites (catecholamine theory)
   – Poor physical health, which weakens emotional coping capacity
   – Medications (particularly phenothiazides, reserpine)
   – Low self-esteem, guilt
   – Anger turned inward
   – Feeling worthless
   – Fear and dependency
   – Unresolved grief

c. **Clinical Manifestations**
   – General lack of interest in life
   – Emotional distress
   – Sadness, pessimism
   – Helplessness, hopelessness
   – Apathy, emptiness
   – Guilt, anxiety
   – Listlessness, fatigue
   – Psychomotor slowing
   – Anorexia, weight loss
   – Constipation
   – Sleep disturbances
   – Loss of libido

d. **Multidisciplinary Approaches**
   – Antidepressant medication
   – Counseling

Additional Nursing Care That Can Be Incorporated into the Generic Care Plan

– Research patient's recent history for a precipitating event or circumstance (death, retirement, relocation, additional financial burden, new medication).
– Evaluate symptoms carefully because they may mimic those of dementia, note any indications of dementia (decline in intellect, personality).
– Offer grief counseling, refer to widow(er)'s group for support if appropriate.
– Suggest new activities, volunteer work to build self-esteem.
– Display positive attitude toward progress, eventual outcome.
– Assist in forming new goals and providing opportunities for success.
– Consult a professional if psychotherapy seems indicated although it tends to be less effective for elderly persons.

- Be alert to and address secondary physical problems such as malnutrition, poor hygiene, constipation, and fatigue.
- Take hints of suicide seriously; the risk is very real; know that attempts may be very subtle (e.g., omitting needed medication, starvation).
- Exercise aggressive observation and supervision if patient has suicidal ideation (see Suicide, page 235).
- Explain to patient that antidepressant medication can take 4–6 weeks before therapeutic effects are experienced.
- Be aware that frequent dosage adjustment may be necessary to achieve maximum benefits from drug therapy and the initial dosage for an older person's usually one-third to one-half the normal adult dosage.
- Instruct patient to continue taking antidepressant medication for several months after improvement is noted.
- Be aware of side effects of antidepressants and evaluate effectiveness of regimen (see Table 9.2).

Table 9.2 Antidepressant Drugs

Examples	Side Effects	Nursing Implications
Tricyclics –Amitriptyline –Desipramine –Doxepin –Imipramine –Nortriptyline –Protriptyline –Tranylcypromine	Dry mouth, diaphoresis, cardiac changes, urinary retention	Offer hard candies, good oral hygiene, fluids. Observe for dehydration, offer fluids, keep skin clean and dry. Obtain baseline and periodic ECG. Monitor vital signs. Monitor I&O.
Trazodone hydrochloride –Desyrel MAO Inhibitors* –Isocarboxazid –Phenelzine sulfate –Tranylcypromine sulfate –Pargyline	Increased or decreased appetite, red eyes, dry mouth, blurred vision, constipation	Administer with food or meals. Observe for drowsiness; administer major dose at bedtime to minimize problems associated with this reaction. Observe serum levels of these drugs as increased levels can occur if administered with digoxin or phenytoin. Monitor vital signs. Advise that positions be changed slowly.
	Indigestion, constipation Toxic symptoms when taken with foods high in tyramine	Ensure adequate nutritional intake, monitor bowel elimination, incorporate foods in diet that will ease digestion and prevent constipation.

(continued)

*MAO inhibitors can have devastating effects on the aged and are not frequently prescribed.

Table 9.2 Antidepressant Drugs (continued)

Examples	Side Effects	Nursing Implications
		Teach patient to avoid foods such as alcohol, chocolate, avocado, yeast extract, pickled herrings, pods of broad beans, chicken livers, and processed or aged cheese.
	Hypotension, drowsiness	Monitor vital signs. Advise that positions be changed slowly. Observe closely.
	Blurred vision, photosensitivity	Supervise activities. Assure safety of environment. Advise to wear sunglasses and use other measures to screen sun.
	Fluctuation of blood glucose level	Monitor blood glucose. Observe for signs of hypoglycemia and hyperglycemia.

Interactions

Increase effects of anticoagulants, atropine-like drugs, antihistamines, sedatives, tranquilizers, narcotics, levodopa.

Decrease effects of clonidine, phenytoin, guanethidine, various antihypertensives.

Effects increased by thiazide diuretics, alcohol.

2. Mania

a. Definition

A mental disorder characterized by a euphoric mood, excessive excitement, and hyperactive behaviors. Many elderly manics have rapid swings between mania and depression, however, less than 10% of all manic-depressive reactions are manic.

b. Etiology

- Affective psychosis
- Meningovascular syphilis
- Medication (stimulants)
- Alcohol
- Psychodynamic

c. **Clinical Manifestations**
   - Elevated mood, elation
   - Accelerated activity
   - Thought processes and speech
   - Reduced sleep requirement
   - Aggressive behavior
   - Irritability
   - Delirium (in severe cases)

d. **Multidisciplinary Approach:**
   Medications (tranquilizers, lithium)

Additional Nursing Care That Can Be Incorporated into the Generic Care Plan

- Minimize stimulation by
  • restricting noise including television and radio, traffic (staff, visitors) and avoiding temperature extremes
  • give short explanations, do not try to explain or reason.
- Meet basic needs by providing foods that can be eaten simply and quickly; a high calorie, high protein diet is beneficial.
- Offer fluids frequently.
- Encourage and allow patient to rest when s/he wishes.
- Protect others from patient and protect patient from humiliating self by controlling bizarre behavior, sexual acting out, etc.
- Monitor blood levels as prescribed for patients receiving lithium since the therapeutic dose is not much less than a toxic dose.
- Be aware that the half-life of lithium is prolonged 50%–100% in the elderly so the initial dose is low and needs to be gradually increased.
- Monitor intake and output because fluid and electrolyte imbalance can promote lithium toxicity.
- Do not restrict sodium intake; many patients are on low salt diets due to cardiac status.

GENERIC CARE PLAN FOR THE NURSING DIAGNOSIS ANXIETY

1. General Information

Anxiety is a state in which the individual experiences feelings of uneasiness, apprehension, and impending doom. The autonomic nervous system is activated in response to a vague, nonspecific threat. Anxiety differs from fear in that the threat is not identifiable.

a. **Etiology**
   - Multiple losses (status, role, possessions, people)
   - Reduced income
   - Loneliness
   - Social isolation, divorce
   - Chronic illness, invasive procedures
   - Change in environment (hospital)
   - Retirement, unemployment

Table 9.3 Antianxiety Drugs

Examples	Side Effects	Nursing Implications
Chlordiazepoxide hydrochloride (Librium) Diazepam (Valium) Hydroxyzine hydrochloride (Vistaril)	Drowsiness, lethargy, weakness, fainting, unsteady gait, confusion, slurred speech, impaired bladder control.	Advise patient to change positions slowly; avoid driving, operating machinery, any activity requiring extreme mental alertness. Supervise activities. Make special effort to understand needs. Keep oriented. Toilet frequently.
Lorazepam (Ativan) Meprobamate (Equinil)	Constipation, nausea, vomiting, GI upset	Maintain adequate fluid and nutrient intake. Monitor nutritional status, I&O.
	Double vision, photosensitivity	Advise on activity limitation. Supervise activities. Use sunglasses, other sunscreen measures.
	Impaired resistance to infection	Observe for and report fever, sore, cellulitis or other signs of infection.
	Dry mouth	Offer hard candies, frequent mouth care.

Interactions: all antianxiety drugs

Increase effects of anticonvulsants, antihypertensives, oral anticoagulants, other CNS depressants.

Effects increased by tricyclic antidepressants.

Combined with anticonvulsants increase seizure activity.

Combined with MAO (monoamine oxidase) inhibitors cause extreme sedation or paradoxical excitement.

b. Clinical Manifestations
  - Physiologic
    - rapid pulse, chest pain, increased blood pressure
    - tremors, trembling, increased psychomotor activity
    - profuse perspiration, cold, clammy hands
    - headaches, dizziness
    - sleep disturbances
    - change in appetite (increased or decreased)
    - change in bowel elimination pattern (increased or decreased)
    - dry mouth, indigestion, nausea
    - urinary frequency
    - aching muscles, tension
    - dyspnea, hyperventilation
  - Cognitive
    - difficulty concentrating, confusion
    - poor memory, forgetfulness
    - narrowed perceptual field, tunnel vision
    - rumination, asking same question repeatedly
    - orientation to past rather than present/future
  - Emotional
    - apprehension
    - helplessness
    - fear/phobias
    - irritability
    - angry outbursts
    - crying
    - losing control
    - criticism of self and others
    - nervousness

c. Multidisciplinary Approaches
  - Antianxiety drugs (see Table 9.3)
  - Psychotherapy

2. Nursing Process

a. Assessment
  - Life situation of family; health, medication history; coping style
  - Recent changes or new stresses (e.g., death of pet, relocation, recently diagnosed illness, reduced income)
  - Level of anxiety and patient's perception of the threat represented by the situation

b. Goal

Patient will recognize anxiety and develop coping mechanisms to reduce and manage anxiety.

c. Interventions

- Eliminate or correct underlying cause if possible (e.g., improve health status, obtain financial aid, help secure home, provide support system).
- Reduce environmental stimuli such as glare and bright lights, noise, and stabilize room temperature; control interruptions and traffic flow.
- Adjust care activities to limit frustration and uncertainty; establish and maintain consistent routines.
- Teach stress-reduction techniques such as deep breathing, visualization, meditation.
- Explain procedures and activities and allow ample time for successful accomplishment.
- Provide simple, repetitive activities to divert attention.
- Offer a warm bath, backrub, or warm milk.
- Encourage expression of feelings and help patient to label feelings of anxiety, etc.
- Minimize patient's responsibilities and decisions.
- Guide patient in finding solutions to problems.
- Assess need for antianxiety medication and give as prescribed; be aware of side effects and interactions (see Table 9.3).
- Be aware that older people require smaller doses of medication; withdraw drugs gradually because they produce physiologic and psychologic dependence.
- Review history for conditions that would contraindicate use of antianxiety drugs (e.g., acute alcohol intoxication; myasthenia gravis; blood dyscrasias; acute narrow-angle glaucoma; severe pulmonary hepatic, or renal disease).

d. Evaluation

- Patient
  • reports a reduction in level of anxiety.
  • develops and uses new coping mechanisms.

e. Possible Related Nursing Diagnoses

Disturbance in self-concept
Impaired social interaction
Ineffective individual coping
Knowledge deficit
Sleep pattern disturbance
Social isolation

GENERIC CARE PLAN FOR THE NURSING DIAGNOSIS
INEFFECTIVE INDIVIDUAL COPING

1. General Information

Ineffective coping is the impairment of adaptive behaviors and problem-solving abilities of a person in meeting life's demands and roles.

a. Etiology
- Situational crises
- Maturational crises
- Unrealistic and/or unmet expectations
- Poor health habits, nutrition, exercise
- Multiple life changes and losses
- Chronic illness
- Inadequate support systems
- Inadequate coping methods

b. Clinical Manifestations
- Destructive behavior toward self or others
- Illness and/or accidents
- Change in communication patterns
- Inability to meet role expectations
- Verbalization of "I can't cope"
- Inability to problem solve
- Excessive smoking, drinking, or drugs
- Insomnia, fatigue
- Irritable, worrying, anxiety, tension
- Frequent complaints of headache, GI symptoms, aches and pains that seem unrelated to any physical problem
- Denial
- Manipulation
- Hostility
- Regression
- Grief

c. Multidisciplinary Approaches
- Address underlying cause if medical (e.g., corrective surgery, fluid and electrolyte replacement)
- Psychotherapy, crisis interventions

2. Nursing Process

a. Assessment
- History for contributing factors (e.g., recent change in life-style, new health problem, added responsibility, loss of significant other)
- Life-long pattern of coping and current functional capacity
- Risks resulting from ineffective coping, such as potential suicide, malnutrition, accidents, victimization, harm to others
- Degree of impairment
- Ability of the patient/family to understand the current situation

b. Goal
Patient and/or family will be able to identify effective strategies to manage stress.

c. Interventions
- Encourage communication with others and converse at patient's level.
- Encourage expression of anxieties, fears, anger, frustration; convey to patient these are normal reactions.
- Assess family health, strengths, weaknesses and relationships to determine members' real ability to assist the patient.
- Address family needs in the care plan; ensure members' ability to assist and cope with long-term patient problems.
- Ensure patient and care givers understand realities of disease and its management.
- Explain procedures prior to doing in a simple, clear manner.
- Use clocks, calendars, pictures, etc., to keep patient oriented to time and place.
- Support patient in evaluating life-style and necessary changes to be made.
- Explore management alternatives with the family to derive acceptable and workable approaches.
- Aid patient in gaining more effective problem solving and stress management techniques
  - discuss how patient can recognize issues and clearly identify the consequences of various actions
  - describe available resources to assist, such as support groups, counselors, hot lines.
- Develop goals; long-term goals give the family a sense of direction and outcome; short-term goals offer milestones upon which to measure progress.
- Teach relaxation exercises and strategies (daily sessions of soft music with eyes closed, yoga, meditation, physical exercise).
- Prioritize care plans to assure that the most pressing patient and family needs are given maximum attention.

d. Evaluation
  – Patient/Family implements
    • effective alternatives to manage stress.
    • coping abilities are identified and utilized.

e. Possible Related Nursing Diagnoses
  Anxiety
  Ineffective family coping
  Potential for injury
  Powerlessness
  Sleep pattern disturbance

Selected Health Problems Frequently Associated with the Nursing Diagnosis INEFFECTIVE INDIVIDUAL COPING

1. Suicide

a. Definition/Discussion
  The act of taking one's own life voluntarily and intentionally. Suicidal behaviors are self-destructive actions that can result in death.
  The elderly have more successful completed attempts of suicide than younger age groups. The peak age for females is between 50–54 years and for males after age 75. The suicide rate is higher for divorced and widowed elderly and double for single men. Suicide rates peak during first year of widowhood and the incidence remains high the first four years.

b. Etiology
  – Depression and factors causing depression
    • widowhood
    • retirement without meaningful role to replace work role
    • relocation (within past 2 years)
    • poverty (primarily those who become poor in old age)
    • social isolation and loneliness
    • physical illness
    • crisis
  – Low impulse control
  – Significant losses incurred
  – Psychiatric problems (psychosis)

c. Clinical Manifestations
  – Purposeful accidents
  – Omission of therapeutic measures

- Self-mutilation
- Depression
- Vague statements about ending one's life
- Alcoholism
- Tunnel vision
- Hostility
- Despair, despondency
- Hopelessness, helplessness
- Grief
- Withdrawal, isolation
- Ambivalence
- Inability to cope

d. Multidisciplinary Approaches
- Antidepressants (see Table 9.2)
- Crisis intervention
- Hospitalization until threat of suicide subsides

Additional Nursing Care That Can Be Incorporated into the Generic Care Plan

- Assess the patient for the level of lethality and the degree of risk to themselves.
- Identify the precipitating event that was the "last straw" for the patient; what happened recently in their life that is different, when did it happen and what is the specific meaning of the event to the individual.
- Assess the person's coping strategies and what has been done in the past when these feelings surface.
- Assess the patient's level of impulse control; presence of excessive drinking or drugs.
- Identify significant others and social resources who can be notified of the patient's suicidal intention.
- Explore past suicide attempts, methods used, and why attempt failed.
- Explore past psychiatric history, chronic illnesses, and previous contacts with counselors, hotlines, etc.
- Explore current life-style, recent losses, and changes.
- Ask patient directly: "Do you have a plan? What is it? When do you plan on carrying it out? Do you have the means to implement your plan?" (pills, gun, etc.).
- Encourage the expression of feelings of hopelessness and despair, give empathy for the situation and reflect back to patient your understanding of the dilemma.
- Realize all suicidal people are ambivalent and appeal to the part of the patient who wants to live.
- Point out to the patient that s/he wants to kill the emotional pain, not him or herself; but that the two are merged in their mind.
- Remove dangerous items from the environment (razor blades, medications, glasses).

- Have someone stay with the patient until the crisis is over.
- Make a verbal or written contract with the patient, stating s/he will call you or someone else (designate who) before a suicide attempt.
- Lend perspective about the problem, give the patient another way to view the situation.
- Identify new coping mechanisms and assist patient in developing constructive ways to manage problem.
- Reinforce positive attributes and behaviors.
- Refer for psychiatric care and support follow up sessions.

2. Alcoholism

a. Definition/Discussion
The abuse, dependency, or addiction to alcohol that threatens physical, emotional, and social health. Older persons are less able to detoxify and excrete alcohol, therefore they are more vulnerable to its effects. Alcoholism decreases ability to cope with age-related physical, mental, and socioeconomic changes. It can increase morbidity and mortality from many otherwise unrelated health problems. Early detection is crucial since the shorter the history of the problem the greater the chance of recovery. It is important that alcoholism be differentiated from other problems causing similar signs, e.g., early dementia, cardiovascular accident. Active intervention can help prevent alcohol abuse among high-risk elderly such as the lonely, depressed, widowed, and poor.

b. Etiology
- Loneliness, depression
- Low self-esteem
- Poor health
- Poor coping abilities
- Dependency traits
- Lifelong pattern
- Familial tendency

c. Clinical Manifestations
- Dependence on alcohol to relieve tension
- Memory blackouts
- Poor nutritional status
- Disrupted personal relationships
- Social isolation
- Arrests for minor violations or driving offenses
- While intoxicated
  - decreased inhibitions
  - clumsiness, staggering
  - mood fluctuation
  - anger, depression

- Signs of related complications
  • gastritis
  • nutritional deficiencies
  • cirrhosis
  • congestive heart failure
  • fluid and electrolyte imbalances
  • hepatitis
  • osteoporosis
  • gastrointestinal bleeding

d. Multidisciplinary Approaches
  - Lab studies to detect alcohol level greater than 150 mg/100 cc
  - Treat concurrent diseases (e.g., cirrhosis, polyneuropathy, pancreatitis)
  - Medications (librium, Antabuse)
  - Psychiatric treatment
  - AA groups, detoxification programs

Additional Nursing Care That Can Be Incorporated into the Generic Care Plan

- Explore drinking history and pattern, amount, frequency, form of alcoholic beverage, precipitating factors, reactions to alcohol, behavioral changes (or the lack of), and alcohol tolerance.
- Observe for withdrawal signs and be aware a decrease in alcohol consumption can cause withdrawal
  • tremors (6–8 hours after last drink)
  • disorientation, hallucination, convulsions (10–30 hours)
  • delirium tremens (60–80 hours).
- Prevent complications during withdrawal (mortality from improperly managed withdrawal is as high as 15%) by
  • administering sedatives (Librium, Valium, other long-lasting CNS depressants) as prescribed
  • monitoring vital signs and general status carefully; an elevated pulse rate could indicate impending delirium tremens
  • gradually withdrawing drugs once patient has stabilized
  • preventing and/or managing seizures by administering magnesium, keeping environment quiet and nonstimulating, maintaining hydration and good nutrition, and offering emotional support.
- Assess for symptoms of possible complications (e.g., jaundice, edema, altered cognition, disorientation, memory deficits, tremors, stupor, pain, congestive heart failure).
- Maintain and improve nutritional status by providing well-balanced meals, supplements, and fluids as
  • Wernicke-Korsakoff syndrome (result of chronic alcoholism) is related to thiamine deficiencies from alcohol
  • polyneuropathy occurs mainly among malnourished alcoholics
  • gastritis and pancreatitis often occur in alcoholics.
- Be knowledgeable of signs and symptoms related to drug interactions

- alcohol interacts with analgesics, antibiotics, anticoagulants, anticonvulsants, antidepressants, antihistamines, barbiturates, digitalis, diuretics, insulin, and iron preparations
- alcohol can cause a tolerance to barbiturates, hypnotics, sedatives, and tranquilizers
- Help patient deal with the underlying reason for drinking.
- Help family and patient to accept diagnosis and support patients efforts to quit.
- Refer to AA, detoxification units, Alanon, and other community resources once the patient accepts that there is a problem with alcohol.

GENERIC CARE PLAN FOR THE NURSING DIAGNOSIS POWERLESSNESS

1. General Information

Powerlessness is a state in which an individual perceives a lack of personal control over certain events or situations. It occurs when one perceives that personal actions will not significantly affect an outcome. These individuals tend to have an external locus of control and believe chance, luck, fate, etc., determine one's life events. The elderly are particularly vulnerable since they have fewer resources, less physical strength, diminished social support and decreased self-esteem all of which increase vulnerability to powerlessness. In addition, psychosocial and physiologic changes inherent in the aging process often lead to an experience of powerlessness. The potential reactions to these feelings can threaten the older person's self-care capacity and quality of life.

a. Etiology
- Illness, particularly those that debilitate or increase dependency
- Sensory deficits
- Psychomotor limitations
- Losses (status, money, support persons)
- Lack of information or skill
- Hospitalization, institutionalization
- Loss of meaningful work/activities
- Stereotyping that denotes inferiority
- Life-style of helplessness

b. Clinical Manifestations
- Expressed feelings of not being in control of situation
- Failure or inability to make decisions
- Apathy, depression
- Aggressive behavior, acting-out, anger, resentment

- Passivity
- Anxiety

c. **Multidisciplinary Approaches:** Psychotherapy

2. Nursing Process

a. **Assessment**
- Underlying cause such as new situation, immobility, illness, lack of knowledge
- Decision-making ability, coping ability, ability to control life, responsibilities
- Effects of powerlessness on total function and well-being
- Locus of control (internal or external)
- Expressions of "giving up" or "no one cares" or a lack of communication
- Manipulative behavior
- Responses to treatments, etc.

b. **Goals**
Patient
- will understand reasons for feeling powerless.
- will identify ways to increase sense of control in own life.

c. **Interventions**
- Eliminate or correct underlying cause, if possible (e.g., provide information, teach new skills, obtain assistive devices).
- Allow maximum control and participation in self-care activities.
- Provide explanations, prepare for procedures.
- Respect patient's desires and decisions.
- Demonstrate concern and caring by listening and encouraging expressions of anger, apathy, and hopelessness.
- Modify the environment to increase patient's control (e.g., call light, telephone, TV within reach).
- Assist patient to set realistic goals and discuss probable outcomes and objectives to reaching desired result.
- Assist patients to maintain an internal locus of control by indicating how events are often determined by one's own behavior; this focus not only gives the person a sense of power, but also inspires hope that there are choices available.
- Give matter-of-fact feedback to patient about manipulative behavior, offer alterative ways to get needs met.
- Assist patient to identify what s/he can do for self.

d. **Evaluation**
   - Patient expresses reduction in feelings associated with powerlessness
   - Patient's control over life activities and decisions is increased.

e. **Possible Related Nursing Diagnoses**
   Disturbance in self-concept
   Ineffective individual coping
   Knowledge deficit
   Sensory-perceptual alterations
   Sleep pattern disturbance
   Social isolation

References

Bartol, M. (1983). Reaching the patient. *Geriatric Nursing, 38*(4), 234.

Beck, A. (1978). *Depression: Causes and treatment.* Philadelphia: University of Pennsylvania Press.

Birren, J., & Sloane, R. (1980). *Handbook of mental health and aging.* Englewood Cliffs, NJ: Prentice-Hall.

Blazer, D. (1982). *Depression in late life.* St. Louis: Mosby.

Feil, N. (1982). *Validation: The Feil method.* Cleveland: Edward Feil Productions.

Gaitz, C. (1983). Identifying and treating depression in an older patient. *Geriatrics, 38*(2), 42–46.

Hall, R. (1984). Tricyclic antidepressants in the treatment of the elderly. *Geriatrics, 39*(4), 81–95.

Jenike, M. (1983). Treating anxiety in elderly patients. *Geriatrics, 38*(10), 115–119.

Kay, P., Waxman, H., & Carner, E. (1983). Detecting psychiatric symptoms in elderly family practice patients. *Gerontologist, 23,* 115.

Lazarus, L. (1982). Brief psychotherapy with the elderly: Process and outcome. *Gerontologist, 22,* 77.

Rosendahl, P., & Ross, V. (1983). Does your behavior affect your patient's response? *Journal of Gerontological Nursing, 9,* 572.

U'Ren, R. (1984). Anxiety, paranoia and personality disorders. In C. Cassel, & G. Walsh (Eds.), *Geriatric medicine, Vol I.* New York: Springer.

Winograd, C. (1984). Mental status tests and the capacity for self-care. *Journal of the American Geriatrics Society, 32*(1), 45–55.

CHAPTER 10

ROLE-RELATIONSHIP
FUNCTIONAL HEALTH PATTERN

A role consists of the behaviors and expectations associated with a particular social position (e.g., spouse, parent, or employee). Roles are learned through a socialization process early in life, thus, an inadequate or unrealistic socialization, or the confrontation of an unfamiliar role, can hinder the adequate fulfillment of roles. For example

- A man who had a father who abused his wife and children may learn this manner of treating his family.
- A woman who has known the role of homemaker throughout her adult life may not understand how to meet the demands of the workplace now that she is widowed and in need of paid employment.

Over the lifespan roles can change because of age (e.g., parent-child relationships), new responsibilities (e.g., remarriage), and increased or decreased status (e.g., loss of income). The major factors influencing the aging person's ability to cope with role changes include

- health status
- experience
- financial resources
- education
- support systems

Role Changes

Parenthood. As children become adults and leave their parental homes parents lose the focus of many of their daily activities. If parents have not developed other sources of activity and fulfillment they may feel a significant loss and stress from this change in their parental role, referred to as the "empty nest syndrome."

With increased age there is greater likelihood that there will be a role reversal. After years of being responsible for their children, parents will become dependent on children for decision making, financial support, and other forms of assistance. This can be a difficult adjustment for both the parents and offspring.

There can also be conflict if adult children remain living in their parents' homes, which more children are doing for longer periods of time. Parents may feel torn between a sense of obligation to their offspring and a desire to be free of daily family responsibilities.

Grandparenthood. A majority of older people are grandparents and they meet this role with a variety of styles. Some grandparents assume an active role in the support, care, and guidance of their grandchildren, while others are remote, visiting only on special occasions and having minimal involvement. For most persons, the grandparent role is more satisfying than stressful; dissatisfaction may result when expectations of grandparents or grandchildren differ from the actual roles assumed.

Retirement. Retirees must adjust to the loss of the job-related sense of purpose, worth, and identity, and to filling large blocks of time. The degree to which these needs are met through other means will determine how successful retirement is.

It is not unusual for a person's early anticipation of retirement to be unrealistic. "Now I can play golf as much as I want." Initially, upon retirement there is excitement as one attempts to fulfill dreams. Eventually this often gives way to boredom and unhappiness with all of the unstructured time. "I don't enjoy golf as much when I can play it whenever I want." Economic constraints may also limit one's fulfillment of dreams. Retirees may need support and counseling to minimize stress and develop meaningful roles to substitute the work role.

Widowhood. The likelihood of becoming widowed increases with each advancing year. For women, widowhood is a greater problem primarily because women tend to marry men older than themselves and women enjoy a longer life expectancy than men. The major factors affecting adjustment to widowhood include cultural background, age, relationship with spouse, financial status, and support systems.

Grief usually is most intense during the first two months after the spouse's death, followed by a year of significant, but less intense, mourning. The widowed person's adjustment should be monitored during this time. The widowhood role solidifies approximately two years after the spouse's death. Widowed persons may need support and guidance in

- developing an identity as a single person
- learning to manage expenses or a household
- adjusting to a reduced income
- exploring new relationships
- establishing sexual relationships
- contemplating remarriage
- organizing life-style

A new, lost, or changed role can be a double-edged sword. It can bring emptiness and devastation or growth and challenge. Individuals need to be viewed in relation to the world in which they interact to fully understand the many facets of their being. Each social position and function draws out different aspects, carries expectations of behavior, and impacts in various ways.

Many of the losses and illnesses of late life can lead to a change in body image, identity, and responses. This can cause the elderly to view themselves negatively and interfere with their social interactions and satisfactory fulfillment of roles and responsibilities. These impairments must be eliminated or minimized to avoid additional risks to health and well-being.

GENERIC CARE PLAN FOR THE NURSING DIAGNOSES
IMPAIRED SOCIAL INTERACTIONS and SOCIAL ISOLATION

1. General Information

Situations of social isolation occur when contact with other people is impaired due to physical, emotional, or socioeconomic factors. A feeling of aloneness develops that can result in other problems and responses such as anxiety, depression, and poor nutrition.

a. Etiology
 – Loss of a relationship: death, relocation, divorce, hospitalization
 – Health problems handicaps, pain, incontinence, emotional illness
 – Poor self-concept disfigurement, obesity, feelings of worthlessness
 – Poverty inability to engage in leisure functions, embarrassment
 – Lack of transportation
 – Sensory losses: poor vision, inability to hear

b. Clinical Manifestations
 – Underactivity
 – Sleep disturbances: excessive or insomnia
 – Appetite disturbances: overeating or anorexia
 – Depression
 – Anxiety, restlessness
 – Anger
 – Inability to concentrate or make decisions
 – Feelings of uselessness, abandonment
 – Desire for more contact, attention seeking
 – Expressed feeling that time is passing slowly

c. Multidisciplinary Approaches
 – Correct or minimize underlying cause, e.g.
   • pain control

- prosthesis, corrective lenses, assistive devices
- psychotherapy
  - Referral to social worker, geriatric activities center, church sponsored activities

2. Nursing Process

a. Assessment
  - Recent changes in health status (e.g., weight gain or loss, fatigue)
  - Possible causative or contributing factors
  - Barriers to social interaction
  - Impact on total health status

b. Goal
Patient will reestablish meaningful social contact and maintain relationships that are supportive and nurturing.

c. Interventions
  - Assist the elderly with adaptation to new roles
    - facilitate open discussion about role changes and how the individual has been affected
    - educate and counsel patient about the realities of the role change linking patient with resources and other persons who share a similar situation
    - help patient find meaningful roles to substitute lost ones or learn skills associated with new roles
    - monitor physical, emotional, and social status to ensure no negative impact by role changes.
  - Eliminate or minimize effects of causative or contributing factors to social isolation
    - introduce new social contacts, senior groups, day-care centers
    - link with resources for transportation, financial aid, telephone reassurance
    - assist in management of medical problems
    - obtain assistive devices to compensate for deficits
    - mobilize family members, friends, neighbors
    - recommend pets, housesharing, alternate housing arrangements
    - recommend participation in a remotivation group (see Table 10.1).
  - Keep in mind that a certain amount of solitude is healthy for all persons; choosing to be alone is different from the inability to have social contact.

d. Evaluation
  - Patient
    - is satisfied with level of social contact
    - is free from secondary problems related to poor social interactions

e. **Possible Related Nursing Diagnoses**
Activity intolerance
Alteration in nutrition
Anxiety
Disturbance in self-concept
Fear
Impaired verbal communication
Powerlessness
Sleep pattern disturbance

GENERIC CARE PLAN FOR THE NURSING DIAGNOSIS
POTENTIAL FOR VIOLENCE

1. General Information

Potential for violence is a state in which the patient is at risk of developing or has demonstrated aggressive behaviors. These behaviors can be a threat to the patient (self-destructive) or to others.

a. **Etiology**
   – Toxic reactions to medications, alcohol
   – Dementias
   – Hormonal imbalances
   – Paranoia, confusion

Table 10.1 Remotivation

Remotivation is a group process to
   –improve grooming and interest in activities of daily living
   –increase interest in world and new activities; mental stimulation
   –increase communication and socialization; ability to discuss topics other than self
    or illness
   –promote self-worth and security through group membership
Group members
   –must have enough cognitive function to participate in structured group activities
    and discussion
   –six to 12 patients meet at regular, prescheduled time, meeting several times a
    week.
Group process
   –Introduce group members and establish a warm, friendly tone.
   –Conduct reality orientation by
    • reviewing current events
    • leading group discussions on such topics as flowers, foreign countries, art
     objects, clothing, school(s), literature
    • eliciting comments, reactions, ideas from *all* members
    • acknowledging *all* contributions.
   –Include an ongoing special activity (e.g., assembling a book, planting a garden,
    planning a trip).
   –Summarize each meeting and express appreciation for members' participation.

- Overwhelming stress
- Fear, misperceptions, response to catastrophic event
- Uncontrolled anger

b. **Clinical Manifestations**
   - Body language, clenched fists, increased motor activity, angry looking facial expression
   - Overt aggressive acts hitting, punching, kicking
   - Evidence of self-injury, bruises, scratches
   - Expressed threats and anger
   - Fear, anxiety, suspiciousness of others or environment

c. **Multidisciplinary Approaches**
   - Treat underlying cause
   - Medications to decrease agitation, anxiety

2. Nursing Process

a. **Assessment**
   - Evidence of violent acts to self and others
   - Life events for possible cause, e.g., new use of alcohol as coping mechanism, bad experiences
   - Complete physical examination to detect physiologic disorders
   - Mental status exam

b. **Goals**
   Patient
   - will gain control over behavior.
   - will learn more constructive ways to express feelings.

c. **Interventions**
   - Discuss behavior with patient; set limits and consequences of exceeding limits of acceptable behavior (e.g., will not be taken on field trip, will be placed in seclusion).
   - Aid patient in developing nonviolent means of expressing feelings (e.g., talking out feelings, walking, physical activity).
   - Control environment to reduce misperceptions and sensory stimuli.
   - Protect patient from harming self and others; observe, remove objects that could be potentially harmful, place in seclusion or restraints if ordered and necessary.
   - Ensure care givers do not respond in aggressive manner or make threats; they need to understand patient's inability to control behavior and importance of calm approach.
   - Adhere to treatment plan to eliminate or minimize underlying cause.

d. Evaluation
– Patient
- is able to control violent behavior.
- experiences elimination or reduction of causative or contributing factors.
- learns new coping behaviors.

e. Possible Related Nursing Diagnoses
Alteration in thought processes
Anxiety
Fear
Ineffective individual coping
Potential for injury
Powerlessness
Sensory-perceptual alteration

References

Bennett, R. (Ed.). (1980). *Aging, isolation and resocialization.* New York: Van Nostrand Reinhold.

Longo, D., & Williams, R. (Eds.). (1978). *Clinical practice in psychosocial nursing assessment and intervention.* New York: Appleton-Century-Crofts.

Rathbone-McCuan, E., & Hashimi, J. (1982). *Isolated elders health and social intervention.* Rockville, MD: Aspen.

Strong, C. (1984). Stress and caring for elderly relatives: Interpretation and coping strategies in an American Indian and White sample. *Gerontologist, 3*(6), 251–256.

CHAPTER 11

SEXUALITY-
REPRODUCTIVE
FUNCTIONAL HEALTH PATTERN

S exuality encompasses more than physical stimulation and pleasure. Sexual identity can determine roles, expectations and self-worth; it can bring pleasure, warmth, and meaning to an older person's life; and offset the many losses that accompany aging.

Sexual function is not normally lost with age, yet attitudes and expectations imply that older adults are not interested in or capable of sex. Few advertisements or media programs portray the elderly as vivacious sexual beings. Older persons who acquire intimate friends or housemates of the opposite sex are often ridiculed or scorned. There is no significant change in sexual attitudes and behaviors with age. Sexual enjoyment neither increases nor decreases. Masturbation, homosexuality, multiple partners, infidelity, and other practices will usually continue in old age.

Institutions are a deterrent to intimacy by separating married couples, discouraging intimate relationships, and reporting residents' sexual behavior to family members. Older couples' privacy is frequently invaded without thought that intimacy may be interrupted.

Sexual responses of the older woman include

- unchanged clitoral response to stimulation
- nipple erections during sexual excitement and possibly several hours after orgasm
- less flushing of the skin (result of a superficial vasocongestive skin response)
- reduced response of labia minoris and majoris
- decreased vaginal lubrication, vaginal wall expansion

251

- similar orgasm and vaginal contractions, although vaginal contractions are of a shorter duration
- urinary frequency and urgency postintercourse.

Sexual responses of the older man include

- erection requires more direct physical stimulation and is more readily lost after interruption
- often able to prolong time before ejaculation
- less flushing of skin
- orgasm is similar to youthful response
- ejaculation may be less forceful, may not occur at all during intercourse (particularly if intercourse is frequent).

GENERIC CARE PLAN FOR THE NURSING DIAGNOSIS
SEXUAL DYSFUNCTION

1. General Information

Sexual dysfunction is an impairment in the ability to experience sexual pleasure.

a. Etiology
  – Male
  - Peyronie's disease: fibrous scarring from chronic inflammation causes painful bending of the penis upon erection
  - prostatitis, other genital infections
    * impotence usually temporary
    * can become permanent with chronic infection
  - spinal trauma
  - medication, particularly antihypertensives and psychotropics
  - prostate surgery (increasingly rare)
  – Female
  - poor lubrication
  - localized infection
  - extended abstinence
  - gynecologic problems: uterine prolapse, rectocele, cystocele
  – Both sexes
  - reduced hormone levels (estrogen, testosterone)
  - social opposition to and/or ridicule of sexual behavior in the elderly
  - illness (self or partner)
    * diabetes mellitus
    * arteriosclerosis
    * Parkinson's disease
    * high blood pressure

* cardiac illness
* arthritis
* neurologic disease
- cosmetic changes (self or partner), altered body function
- boredom, fatigue
- psychologic problems
  * depression
  * stress
  * anxiety
- lack of privacy
- unavailability of partner, prolonged sexual inactivity
- negative personal attitude toward sex (may have never found sex pleasurable or had some bad experience)
- poor self-esteem, psychosocial abuse
- lack of knowledge
- high intake of alcohol, overeating
- pain, joint inflexibility

b. Clinical Manifestations
  - Male: impotence
  - Female: dyspareunia (painful intercourse)
  - Verbalization of problem in sexuality
  - Frequent seeking of confirmation of desirability

c. Multidisciplinary Approaches
  - Improvement of underlying problem (weight reduction, pain control)
  - Sexual counseling
  - Psychotherapy

2. Nursing Process

a. Assessment
Review of sexual function as part of the overall evaluation of all elderly clients.
  - Review lifelong sexual activity (helps place patient's current condition into perspective)
  - Females: menstrual/pregnancy history, sexual interest/activity, pattern of gynecologic care (professional visits and self-examination), genitalia, breasts
  - Males: sexual interest/activity, genitalia, prostate
  - Impact of illness or surgery on sexuality; changes in roles, lowered self-esteem
  - Knowledge level, misinformation

b. Goal

Client will achieve desired satisfaction in the expression of own sexuality.

c. Interventions

− Set an accepting, nonjudgmental, and open tone when discussing sexual problems with older persons.
− Encourage open expression and discussion of sexual concerns.
− Assist in resolving sexual problems by
  • counseling and educating as necessary
  • arranging for comprehensive examination if an organic problem is suspected
  • discussing realistic limitations in the face of illness
  • seeking resources from organizations to help clients compensate for disease-related sexual limitations (e.g., the Arthritis Foundation has literature demonstrating alternate sexual positions for patients with severe symptoms)
  • referring to sex counselors and clinics if specific therapy is indicated.
− Educate the patient about real sexual changes accompanying age; discount myths.
− Stress physical care in maintenance of sexual function
  • genital hygiene
  • regular medical examination (gynecologic/prostate)
  • self-examination (breast, penis)
  • prevention/recognition of infections, complications of chronic diseases.
− Reinforce patient's sexual identity by acknowledging and assisting with efforts to look attractive.
− Respect the privacy of patients, provide for uninterrupted time alone to be with partner.
− Treat intimate relationships among older persons with dignity and seriousness.
− Be alert to patients and significant others comments and behavior that may indicate a concern regarding sexual functioning or satisfaction.

d. Evaluation

− Patient
  • resumes ability to obtain sexual pleasure
  • learns alternative means of obtaining sexual gratification

e. Possible Related Nursing Diagnoses

Alteration in family processes
Anxiety
Impaired social interaction

Selected Health Problems Frequently Associated with the Nursing Diagnosis SEXUAL DYSFUNCTION

1. Breast Cancer

a. Definition

A malignant growth within breast tissue and a leading cause of cancer deaths in the elderly. Decreased fat and atrophy of the breasts with age may make masses more evident in later life. Although a problem primarily affecting women, nearly 2% of all breast cancers occur in men.

b. Etiology
- Cause unknown
- Predisposing factors are
  - family history of breast cancer
  - nulliparity
  - late menopause

c. Clinical Manifestations
- Nontender lump
- Recently developed asymmetry of breasts
- Dimpling, "orange-peel" skin
- Nipple discharge
- Bleeding
- Retraction
- Palpable nodular masses
- Signs of advanced disease
  - pain
  - weight loss
  - weakness

d. Multidisciplinary Approaches
- Diagnostic tests
  - mammography
  - thermography
  - xerography
  - biopsy
- Surgery: Segmental resection, modified or radical mastectomy
- Radiation, chemotherapy, hormonal manipulation

Additional Nursing Care That Can Be Incorporated into the Generic Care Plan

– Instruct all female clients in monthly breast self-examination; link examination date to regular monthly event (e.g., when the social security check is received or the electric bill paid).
– Recommend annual mammography.
– Obtain prompt medical evaluation when suspicious mass or breast change is discovered.
– Ensure patient understands treatment alternatives if malignancy is present.
– If surgery is performed
  • observe for complication of lymphedema of arm (e.g., swelling of arm on operative side)
  • initiate rehabilitative measures such as exercises to promote full range of motion to arm and shoulders
  • arrange for prosthesis as soon as possible.
– Offer emotional support to patient and husband
  • encourage ventilation of feelings
  • clarify misconceptions
  • link with support group (e.g., Reach to Recovery).
– Reinforce importance of regular follow-up.

2. Senile Vaginitis

a. Discussion
Common among older women because of age-related changes, e.g., gradual atrophy of vaginal tissues, decrease in vaginal lubrication, size of uterus and cervix, that predispose to infection.

b. Etiology
– Age-related changes
– Trauma
– Poor hygiene

c. Clinical Manifestations
– Vaginal itching
– Soreness, burning
– Redness, discharge

d. Multidisciplinary Approaches
– Local medications to treat specific organism
– Acid douches

Additional Nursing Care That Can Be Incorporated into the Generic Care Plan

- Question and educate patient at risk (many older women view vaginitis as a younger woman's problem and may not associate their symptoms with it).
- Instruct in proper hygiene.
- Reinforce treatment plan
  - do not assume patient understands that topical medications should not be ingested; give specific instructions
  - if douche is prescribed, emphasize importance of measuring water temperature to prevent burning to fragile vaginal tissue

3. Impotency

a. Definition
Impotency is an inability to obtain a penile erection. It can be temporary or permanent, and result from either organic or psychologic causes. Impotency is not normal.

b. Etiology
- Depression, anxiety
- Drugs (particularly antihypertensives)
- Obesity
- Alcoholism
- Diabetes
- Neurologic disorders

c. Clinical Manifestations
- Partial or complete inability of penis to become erect

d. Multidisciplinary Approaches
- Penile implant
- Counseling
- Treat underlying cause
- Encourage patient to obtain a thorough evaluation of the problem.

Additional Nursing Care That Can Be Incorporated into the Generic Care Plan

- Ensure patient understands realities of condition; counsel as to whether or not returned potency can be anticipated.
- Assist patient and partner in achieving sexually satisfying relationship
  - emphasize importance of patience and continuing efforts
  - discuss forms of sexual gratification other than intercourse (touching, oral sex, masturbation)

• discuss the role of performance anxiety and how it effects one's physiologic responses.
– Refer to a sex therapist if patient desires to deal with the situation more in depth.

References

Butler, R., & Lewis, M. (1976). *Sex after sixty.* New York: Harper and Row.
Damrosch, S. (1984). Graduate nursing students' attitudes toward sexually active older persons. *Gerontologist, 24*(3), 299–302.
Eliopoulos, C. (1984). Assessment of sexual function. In C. Eliopoulos (Ed.), *Health assessment of the older adult.* Menlo Park, CA: Addison-Wesley.
Kaas, M. (1978). Sexual expression of the elderly in nursing homes. *Gerontologist, 18*(4), 372–378.
Labby, D. (1984). Sexuality. In C. Cassel, & J. Walsh (Eds.), *Geriatric medicine (Vol II.)* New York: Springer.

CHAPTER 12

VALUE-BELIEF
FUNCTIONAL HEALTH PATTERN

M ost individuals possess a set of beliefs that guide their lives. These beliefs give a reason for existence, hope, and a sense of right and wrong. One's attitudes toward growing old and managing health and illness can be influenced by the beliefs held. For example, a different level of acceptance accompanies a belief that the ills of the aged are God's will and must be accepted than would exist if one believed individuals control their own destinies and must use every resource available to fight illness.

Values and beliefs do not dissolve when a person becomes aged or ill. In fact, they may become more important than ever. Nurses must be familiar with various religious beliefs and philosophies so that they may respect, advocate, and support practices consistent with them.

Facing Death

As aging people witness increasing numbers of contemporaries dying and experience more health problems themselves they become acutely aware of their own mortality. Such an awareness that death is a reality and may soon be approaching often stimulates older persons to evaluate the meaning of their lives. There may be an interest in putting their lives in order, resolving conflicts with family and friends, planning for the distribution of estates, and assuring the well-being of loved ones. Individuals' lifelong patterns of dealing with problems will influence how they confront the recognition that their years of life are shrinking. The pragmatic father who began his child's college fund before that child was born may have developed a detailed will describing the disposition of all his assets and his preferences for terminal care, while the person who lived one day at a time and retreated from problems may not give any consideration to his/her own mortality. There is no single style of confronting death. People will die as they have lived.

A terminal illness makes death an inescapable reality. This profound experience may trigger a variety of emotional reactions. Dr. Elizabeth Kübler-

Ross in her book *On Death and Dying* (1970) categorized these reactions into the stages of denial, anger, bargaining, depression, and acceptance (see Table 12.1). Not all dying persons experience every stage, nor will they progress through the stages in an orderly manner. Family members and care givers, also, may experience similar reactions as they cope with the loss of the dying person. Engel (1964) identifies the bereavement phases for survivors as shock, developing awareness of loss, and restitution.

The realization that death is imminent can be devastating and emotionally crippling if one feels life has been useless or insignificant. By helping the elderly to evaluate their lives, nurses can help older patients to work through unresolved feelings and recognize accomplishments. The result can be enhanced self-esteem, satisfaction with one's life, and a clearer understanding of the "unfinished business" that needs to be resolved in one's remaining life.

The process of *life review* has been described as an essential part of letting go and preparing for death (Butler and Lewis, 1982). Nurses can support efforts of life review by promoting reminiscence by older adults, either individually or through group activity (see Table 9.1).

Reminiscence may not be a comfortable experience for patients or nurses. It can be difficult to rekindle old anger, frustrations, guilt, disappointments, and other feelings; a variety of reactions can result. Nurses must understand that these uncomfortable reactions may need to be experienced to resolve past conflicts. Patients need support during this experience and reassurance that they managed situations in the best manner that they could at the time.

Table 12.1   Emotional Reactions to Dying

Denial:	By avoiding the topic of death the patient can gain time to mobilize defenses. It is important to allow the patient this time and not force discussions regarding the terminal nature of the illness or death.
Anger:	Hostility and rage are felt as the patient begins to think about the reality of death and experience bitterness that it is happening. Frequently, family and staff closest to the patient receive this displaced anger. The patient needs to release tension by venting this feeling and the most helpful approach for nurses is to accept this anger without judgment or being personally hurt.
Bargaining:	The patient may try to extend life by seeking compromises or "trade-offs." Many times, bargaining is done through prayers. Support is needed during this period, as well as protection that the patient doesn't get taken advantage of by quacks and others who offer unrealistic cures or life extensions.
Depression:	A form of mourning occurs as the patient considers the losses which will be faced. The patient will need support and the presence of others—even if this means sitting in silence for extended periods of time. Human contact through hand holding and massages can be especially helpful.
Acceptance:	As the patient comes to terms with death he or she may be able to discuss it and begin to address issues openly. Support is needed as the patient openly expresses feelings and discusses plans.

(Kübler-Ross, 1969)

Strengths and accomplishments should be reinforced, and shortcomings need to be forgiven. The more the individual can accept the totality of his/her life, the successes and failures, the more integration occurs and the less despair one feels. Acceptance of choices and life as lived is the key to inner peace.

GENERIC CARE PLAN FOR THE NURSING DIAGNOSIS
SPIRITUAL DISTRESS

1. General Information

Spiritual distress is a state in which beliefs or value systems are disturbed, or at risk of being disturbed. Illness, multiple losses, and facing death require the individual to rely upon his or her spiritual beliefs and practices to maintain the strength and courage to continue living. When people begin to question "Why me?" and "What's the meaning of this event?" they are experiencing a conflict between their beliefs and the reality of the situation. Spiritual distress results. The individual's beliefs and values no longer provide a framework for understanding life and one's purpose and place here on earth. Nurses need to promote spiritual integrity to strengthen the patient's ability to manage life's challenges and problems, and to give meaning to life.

a. Etiology
- Physical illness
  - altered body image
  - loss of function
  - pain
- Terminal illness
- Change in meaningful relationships
  - illness or loss of significant other
  - own limitation in continuing relationship
- Limitations imposed by situation or others
  - hospitalization, institutionalization
  - isolation, confinement
  - opposition or interference by care givers, family
- Conflicts between religious practices and prescribed treatment
  - special diet
  - medications, transfusions, IVs
  - life-sustaining measures

b. Clinical Manifestations
- Anger, resentment over suffering, meaning of life
- Anxiety, fear
- Guilt
- Unable to practice usual religious rituals

- Discouragement
- Verbalizes doubts or concerns about beliefs
- Requests visit from clergy
- Questioning ("Why me? Why now?") credibility of belief system

c. **Multidisciplinary Approaches**
- Possible alteration of treatment plan to be consistent with beliefs
- Pastoral counseling

2. Nursing Process

a. **Assessment**
- Religious beliefs, practices, preferences
  - determine type of belief, e.g., God, Buddha, man is in control of his own destiny (see Table 12.2)
  - desires to have any specific member of clergy or religious organization contacted
  - what measures can assist in supporting religious practices, e.g., taking to chapel Sunday mornings, obtaining a Bible, providing 15 minutes privacy each morning
- Beliefs that could conflict with health practices or treatment plan, e.g., refusal of medications, dietary practices

b. **Goal**
Patient will maintain religious beliefs and practices to maximum degree possible.

c. **Interventions**
- Acquaint all care givers with patient's needs and desires pertaining to religious beliefs; ensure care givers are nonjudgmental.
- Make necessary arrangements for continuation and support of religious practices (e.g., obtain special articles, arrange for clergy visitation, pray with patient or arrange for someone else to).
- Adhere to imposed practices or restrictions unless the patient has decided to violate them.
- Obtain dietary consultation or arrange for special foods to be brought from home.
- Avoid shaving beards if against Orthodox practice.
- Know specific Sabbath days and respect them.
- Follow unique postmortem practices.
- Allow patient to express feelings; understand that life review and a discussion of the reasons for current problems aid in putting one's life in perspective and understanding its purpose.

d. **Evaluation**
- Patient's spiritual beliefs and practices are maintained to maximum extent possible.

Table 12.2   Impact of Religious Beliefs on Health Practices

Religion	Special Dietary Practices	Unique View of Illness	Treatment Beliefs	Practices Related to Death
Baptist	No alcohol, coffee, tea, pork, tobacco	Form of punishment; Satan's work	Divine healing through laying on of hands; some resistance to medical treatment	May desire communion
Buddhist	Vegetarian, no alcohol or tobacco	Test of strength to aid in development of soul	May oppose medications, desire for cleanliness; no treatment on holy days	May desire last rites by Buddhist priest
Catholic	Fast from meats on Ash Wednesday and Good Friday; optional on Fridays and during Lent	Allowed by God because of man's sins although not believed to be a form of God's punishment	Modern medical treatment; confession and Communion may be desired	Last rites by priest
Church of Christ	Same as Baptist			
Church of Christ, Scientist		Result of negative or faulty thoughts	Oppose medications, IVs, transfusions, physical exams, psychotherapy, assistance from health professionals; use treatments by specific Christian Science practitioners	May desire support from Christian Science reader
Church of God	Same as Baptist			
Episcopal	No meat on Fridays, fast during Lent and prior to Communion		Spiritual healing	May desire confession, Communion, last rites
Friends (Quakers)	No alcohol	Acceptance	May resist use of drugs	Do not believe in afterlife; individual relates to God without priests or ministers
Greek Orthodox	Fast during Lent and before Communion	May desire anointment and Communion to manage illness	Support measures to maintain life	May desire communion and last rites by priest

(continued)

Table 12.2 Impact of Religious Beliefs on Health Practices (continued)

Religion	Special Dietary Practices	Unique View of Illness	Treatment Beliefs	Practices Related to Death
Hindu	Vegetarian, no alcohol	May result from sins from previous life	May believe in self-management and control of illness; cleanliness important	Thread tied around neck or wrist by priest; water put in mouth; family cleanses body after death; support cremation
Jehovah's Witness	Do not eat meats containing blood; meats must be drained	Manage without modern interventions	Against modern treatment, including transfusions	
Judaism	May follow kosher diet; fast on Yom Kippur and Tisha Bab; use matzo instead of leavened bread during Passover		Supports modern medical treatment; may refuse care on Sabbath	Do not believe in afterlife; religious persons wash body after death; body buried as soon as possible
Lutheran			Supports modern medical treatment; may want Communion or blessing by minister	May desire last rites
Mennonite			May resist medications	
Mormon	No tea, coffee, alcohol, tobacco; may limit meat intake	Results from violation of God's commandments or laws of health	Divine healing through laying on of hands; may oppose medical treatment	Baptism of deceased; may preach to the deceased
Muslim	No pork, alcohol; may fast during Ramadan	God's will	Accept treatments if not in violation of practices; cleanliness important	Confession prior to death; family prepares body after death; body must face Mecca
Pentecostal	Same as Baptist			
Presbyterian	Same as Lutheran			
Russian Orthodox	Same as Greek Orthodox			

Table 12.2   Impact of Religious Beliefs on Health Practices (continued)

Religion	Special Dietary Practices	Unique View of Illness	Treatment Beliefs	Practices Related to Death
Scientologist		Health affected by thinking, beliefs	May oppose psychiatric treatment	May desire confession or visit with pastoral counselor
Seventh-day Adventist	No coffee, tea, alcohol; some may not eat meat and shellfish		May believe in divine healing; treatment may be opposed on Sabbath	May desire baptism or communion
Unitarian		Believe in individual's responsibility for health status	Modern medical treatment	Support cremation

Note: From "Spiritual Distress" by L. Carpenito, 1983, *Nursing diagnosis application to clinical practice*, pp. 453–462. Philadelphia: Lippincott. (Reprinted with permission.)

e. **Possible Related Nursing Diagnoses**
Anxiety
Fear
Grieving
Hopelessness
Ineffective coping
Knowledge deficit
Powerlessness
Sleep pattern disturbance

GENERIC CARE PLAN FOR THE NURSING DIAGNOSIS GRIEVING

1. General Information

Grief is the emotional reaction that follows the loss of a love object. The duration of the reaction varies but may last for over a year. Grief disrupts daily life and often affects physical functioning as well. The elderly not only experience numerous losses but are required to face the inevitability of death.

a. Etiology
- Loss of health, energy, activity
- Loss of role related to family, job
- Loss of financial income, altered economic status
- Loss of youth and beauty, life
- Loss of friends, family, spouse
- Loss of home, alterations in living accommodations
- Loss of mobility, senses
- Diagnosis of a terminal illness

b. Clinical Manifestations
- Somatic symptoms
  - fatigue, insomnia
  - empty feelings, lump in the throat
  - hyperventilation
  - anorexia
- Psychologic symptoms
  - shock, disbelief, denial, avoidance
  - anger, mental discomfort, irritability
  - bargaining, loss of faith "why me?"
  - sorrow, crying, depression
- Behavioral symptoms
  - complaining, demanding
  - hostility, rage, bitterness
  - displaced anger on to staff, family
  - avoidance of feelings by using distractions (e.g., TV, busywork)
  - discouragement, "giving up"

c. Multidisciplinary Approaches
- Counseling, religious referral
- Group support
- Medication for anxiety, depression

2. Nursing Process

a. Assessment
- Exact nature of the losses and when they occurred
- Meaning of the loss to the individual
- Realistic perception of losses or potential loss
- Social and cultural perceptions of the meaning of death, life after death, and how to prepare for death
- Spiritual beliefs and practices; desire for religious counsel
- Stage of grief
- Physical reactions, need for assistance in activities of daily living
- Available support system

b. **Goal**

Patient will be able to cope with the losses or the impending death by adaptively completing each stage of the grief and mourning process.

c. **Interventions**

- Encourage open expression of feelings but don't force discussion beyond what the patient is willing to face.
- Encourage hope, assist patient in making plans, but do not foster unrealistic goals and beliefs.
- Answer questions honestly, provide information about present status as needed.
- Be aware that the patient may insist upon second and third opinions about prognosis, or claim there is a mix up; this is part of the denial phase.
- Allow denial as long as necessary since it allows the patient to mobilize personal defenses.
- Be sensitive to changing emotional states; patient may fluctuate between one stage and another.
- Recognize the stages of anger and bargaining and how they manifest themselves; displaced feelings, "why me?", trying to secure more time to finish business.
- Do not take patient's anger toward staff personally; displacement of anger and frustrations is a common occurrence.
- Provide comfort, physical contact, and frequent interactions.
- Pay particular attention to physical needs; feed if necessary, provide protection and comfort, introduce preventive measures to maintain nutrition and elimination patterns.
- Give medication as needed for pain, anxiety, depression.
- Be alert to new physical and emotional symptoms and evaluate relation to stage of grief.
- Be sensitive to the emotional needs of family and friends, suggest counseling if appropriate.
- Prepare patient and family for the inevitable depression that follows recognition that all attempts at bargaining are futile, and one has to accept the loss of relationships, unfulfilled dreams and life itself.
- Allow time to spend with patient discussing how s/he is preparing for death, saying goodbye to people, things, life, etc.
- Encourage patients to resolve "unfinished business" and conflicts with loved ones; plan disposition of their estate and make a will.
- Recognize the problem of loneliness for elderly people and their ambivalent desire to end the pain and isolation versus the instinctive desire to live and the fear of death.
- Assist the family in funeral preparation by referring to appropriate resources for arrangements, insurances, social security benefits, etc.

- Assist family in ventilating feelings and continue to support family after patient's death.
- Suggest professional help for anyone suffering from dysfunctional grief.

d. Evaluation
- Patient
  • adapts constructively to losses incurred.
  • is able to speak realistically about loss with an acceptance of the consequences.
  • exhibits minimal denial, anger and sorrow.

e. Possible Related Nursing Diagnoses
Alteration in family processes
Anxiety, fear
Hopelessness
Ineffective individual coping
Sleep pattern disturbance
Spiritual distress

References

Albert, M., & Steffl, B. (1984). Loss, grief, and death in old age. In B. Steffl (Ed.), *Handbook of gerontological nursing.* New York: Van Nostrand Reinhold.
Butler, R. and Lewis, M. (1982). *Aging and mental health* (3rd ed.). St. Louis: Mosby.
Carpenito, L. (1983). *Nursing diagnosis application to clinical practice.* Philadelphia: Lippincott.
Engel, G. (1964). Grief and grieving. *American Journal of Nursing, 64,* 93–98.
Erikson, E. (1963). *Childhood and society* (2nd ed.). New York: W. W. Norton.
Fisher, R. (1983). Management of the dying elderly patient. *Journal of the American Geriatrics Society, 31*(9), 563–564.
Hershkowitz, M. (1984). To die at home: Rejection of medical intervention by geriatric patients who had serious organic disease. *Journal of the American Geriatrics Society, 32*(6), 457–459.
Kübler-Ross, E. (1969). *On death and dying.* New York: Macmillan.
Lund, D. (1984). Can pets help the bereaved? *Journal of Gerontological Nursing, 10*(6), 8–12.
Marshall, J. (1983). The dying patient. In W. Reichel (Ed.), *Clinical aspects of aging* (2nd ed.). Baltimore: Williams & Wilkins.
Marshall, J. (1983). The dying elderly patient, *American Family Physician, 28*(5), 161–165.
Peck, R. (1956). Psychological development in the second half of late life. In J. Anderson (Ed.), *Psychological aspects of aging.* Washington, DC: American Psychological Association.
Watson, W., & Maxwell, R. (Eds.). (1977). *Human aging and dying.* New York: St. Martin's Press.

APPENDIX A
STANDARDS FOR GERONTOLOGIC NURSING PRACTICE

Standard I
Data are systematically and continuously collected about the health status of the older adult. The data are accessible, communicated, and recorded.

Standard II
Nursing diagnoses are derived from the identified normal responses of the individual to aging and the data collected about the health status of the older adult.

Standard III
A plan of nursing care is developed in conjunction with the older adult and/or significant others that includes goals derived from the nursing diagnosis.

Standard IV
The plan of nursing care includes priorities and prescribed nursing approaches and measures to achieve the goals derived from the nursing diagnosis.

Standard V
The plan of care is implemented, using appropriate nursing actions.

Standard VI
The older adult and/or significant other(s) participate in determining the progress attained in the achievement of established goals.

Standard VII
The older adult and/or significant other(s) participate in the ongoing process of assessment, the setting of new goals, the reordering of priorities, the revision of plans for nursing care, and the initiation of new nursing actions.

APPENDIX B
REFERENCE FOR LABORATORY VALUES

Hematocrit

Men	*Women*
38%-54%	35%-47%

Hemoglobin

Men	*Women*
14-18 gm/100 cc	12-16 gm/100 cc

Sedimentation Rate

Men	*Women*
< 20 mm/hour	< 30 mm/hour

Blood Cells

Constituent	Normal Values	Deviations
Red blood cells		Increase
Men	4,600,000-6,200,000/mm^3	– Acute poisoning
Women	4,200,000-5,400,000/mm^3	– Bone marrow hyperplasia
		– Dehydration
		– Diarrhea
		– Polycythemia
		– Pulmonary fibrosis
		Decrease
		– Anemias
		– Hemorrhage
		– Hypothyroidism
		– Thalassemia
		– Toxicity
White blood cells	5,000-10,000/mm^3	Increase
		– Acute bacterial infection
		– Leukemia
		– Polycythemia
		Decrease
		– Acute alcohol ingestion
		– Acute viral infection
		– Agranulocytosis
		– Bone marrow depression

Blood Cells (continued)

Constituent	Normal Values	Deviations
Neutrophils	50%-70% of total WBC Count	Increase – Acute hemorrhage – Bacterial infections – Carcinoma – Cushing's disease – Diabetes mellitus – Gout – Hemolytic anemia – Increased corticosteroids – Lead poisoning – Pancreatitis – Rheumatic fever – Rheumatoid arthritis – Thyroiditis – Stress Decrease – Acute viral infection – Bone marrow damage – Folic acid deficiency – Vitamin B_{12} deficiency
Eosinophils	1%-4% of total WBC Count	Increase – Allergy – Colitis – Collagen diseases – Eosinophilic granulomatosis – Eosinophilic leukemia – Parasitosis
Basophils	0%-1% of total WBC Count	Increase – Myelofibrosis – Polycythemia vera Decrease – Anaphylactic reaction
Lymphocytes	20%-40% of total WBC Count	Increase – Cushing's disease – Infectious diseases – Leukemia – Thyrotoxicosis
Monocytes	0%-6% of total WBC Count	Increase – Malaria – Subacute bacterial endocarditis – Tuberculosis – Typhoid fever

Blood Cells (continued)

Constituent	Normal Values	Deviations
Platelets	200,000-350,000/mm³	Increase – Chronic granulocytic leukemia – Hemoconcentration – Polycythemia – Splenectomy Decrease – Acute leukemia – Aplastic anemia – Bone marrow depression – Chemotherapy – Thrombocytopenic purpura

Blood Chemistry

Constituent	Normal Values	Deviations
Bilirubin, Total	0.1-1.2 mg/100 cc	Increase – Liver disease – Hemolysis post transfusion – Pernicious anemia – (Jaundice present when bilirubin level exceeds 1.5 mg/100 cc) Decrease – Carcinoma – Chronic renal disease
Calcium	9-11 mg/100 cc (4.5-5.5 mEq/liter)	Increase – Addison's disease – Hyperparathyroidism – Malignant bone tumors Decrease – Chronic renal disease – Hypoparathyroidism – Vitamin D deficiency
Bicarbonate	(24-32 mEq/liter)	Increase – Alkalosis – Intestinal obstruction – Respiratory disease – Tetany – Vomiting Decrease – Acidosis

Blood Chemistry

Constituent	Normal Values	Deviations
Bicarbonate–(continued)		Decrease – Diarrhea – Nephritis
Chloride	350-390 mg/100 cc (95-105 mEq/liter)	Increase – Renal tubular acidosis Decrease – Diuretics which save potassium – Hypokalemic alkalosis – Ingestion of potassium without chloride – Loss of gastric secretions
Cholesterol Total Free Esterified	 150-250 mg/100 cc 40-50 mg/100 cc 75-210 mg/100 cc	Increased – Chronic renal disease – Diabetes mellitus – Hypothyroidism – Liver disease with jaundice – Pancreatic dysfunction Decrease – Fasting state – Hemolytic anemia – Hypermetabolic states – Hyperthyroidism – Intestinal obstruction – Liver disease – Malnutrition – Pernicious anemia – Tuberculosis
Creatinine	0.6-1.2 mg/100 cc	Increase – Chronic glomerulonephritis – Nephrosis – Pyelonephritis – Other renal dysfunctions
Fibrinogen	150-300 mg/100 cc	Increase – Infection Decrease – Liver disease – Malnutrition
Glucose	70-120 mg/100 cc	Increase – Cerebral lesions – Cushing's disease

Blood Chemistry (continued)

Constituent	Normal Values	Deviations
		– Diabetes mellitus
		– Emotional stress
		– Exercise
		– Hyperthyroidism
		– Infections
		– Pancreatic dysfunctions
		– Steroid therapy
		– Thiazide diuretic therapy
		Decrease
		– Addison's disease
		– Beta cell neoplasm
		– Hyperinsulinism
		– Hypothyroidism
		– Starvation
Iodine, protein-bound	4-8 mcg/100 cc	Increase
		– Hyperthyroidism
		Decrease
		– Hypothyroidism
Iron	65-170 mcg/100 cc	Increase
		– Aplastic anemia
		– Hemolytic anemia
		– Hemochromatosis
		– Hepatitis
		– Pernicious anemia
		Decrease
		– Iron deficiency anemia
Lead	< 40 mcg/100 cc	Increase
		– Lead poisoning
Lipids, Total	400-1000 mg/100 cc	Increased
		– Diabetes mellitus
		– Glomerulonephritis
		– Hypothyroidism
		– Nephrosis
		Decrease
		– Hyperthyroidism
pCO_2 *(arterial)*	35-45 mm Hg	Increase
		– Metabolic alkalosis
		– Respiratory acidosis
		Decrease
		– Metabolic acidosis
		– Respiratory alkalosis
pH *(arterial)*	7.35-7.45	Increase
		– Fever

Blood Chemistry (continued)

Constituent	Normal Values	Deviations
Ph–(continued)		Increase − Hyperapnea − Intestinal obstruction − Vomiting Decrease − Diabetic acidosis − Hemorrhage − Nephritis − Uremia
Phosphatase Acid Alkaline	0.5-3.5 units 2-4.5 units	Increase − Bony metastasis − Carcinoma of the prostate

pO₂ (arterial)	95-100 mm Hg	Increase
		− Administration of
		  pure O_2
		Decrease
		− Circulatory disorders
		− Decreased hemoglobin
		− Decreased O_2 supply
		− High altitudes
		− Poor O_2 uptake and
		  utilization
		− Respiratory exchange
		  problems

Potassium	18-22 mg/100 cc (3.5-5.5 mEq/liter)	Increase − Addison's disease − Anuria − Bronchial asthma − Burns − Renal disease − Tissue breakdown − Trauma Decrease − Cirrhosis − Cushing's disease − Diabetic acidosis − Diarrhea − Diuretic therapy − Potassium-free intravenous therapy − Steroid therapy − Vomiting

Blood Chemistry (continued)

Constituent	Normal Values	Deviations
Protein, Total	6-8 gm/100 cc	Increase – Infections Decrease – Intestinal tract disease – Liver disease – Malnutrition – Renal disease
Protein, Albumin	3.2-4.5 gm/100 cc	Increase – Multiple myeloma Decrease – Acute stress – Chronic infection – Chronic liver disease – Loss of plasma – Malabsorption of protein – Malnutrition – Nephrotic syndrome
Protein, Globulin	2.3-3.5 gm/100 cc	Increase – Chronic hepatitis – Chronic infections – Collagen disease – Leukemia – Liver disease – Multiple myeloma – Sarcoidosis Decrease – Proteinuria
Sodium	310-340 mg/100 cc (135-145 mEq/liter)	Increase – Cardiac disease – Cushing's disease – Cirrhosis – Congestive heart failure – Dehydration – Diabetic acidosis – Diarrhea – Diuretic therapy – Excessive ingestion of water – Overhydration intravenously – Starvation

Blood Chemistry (continued)

Constituent	Normal Values	Deviations
Urea nitrogen *(BUN)*	10-18 mg/100 cc	Increase – Acute glomerulonephritis – Burns – Dehydration – Gastrointestinal hemorrhage – High protein intake – Intestinal obstruction – Mercury poisoning – Prostatic hypertrophy – Protein catabolism – Renal disease Decrease – Cirrhosis – Liver disease – Low protein intake – Starvation
Uric acid Men Women	2.1-7.8 mg/100 cc 2-6.4 mg/100 cc	Increase – Chronic lymphocytic and granulocytic leukemia – Chronic renal failure – Fasting – Gout – High salicylate intake – Leukemia – Multiple myeloma – Pneumonia – Thiazide diuretic therapy Decrease – Allopurinol therapy

Urine Chemistry

Constituent	Normal Values	Deviations
Acetone; *Acetoacetate*	0	Increase – Starvation – Uncontrolled diabetes
Creatine	0-200 mg/24 hour	Increase – Fever – Hyperthyroidism – Liver cancer

Urine Chemistry (continued)

Constituent	Normal Values	Deviations
Creatinine	0.8-2 gm/24 hour	Increase – Salmonella infections – Tetanus – Typhoid fever Decrease – Anemia – Leukemia – Muscular atrophy – Renal failure
Creatinine clearance	100-150 cc/min	Decrease – Renal disease
Glucose	Negative (1 + not unusual finding in older adults)	Increase – Diabetes mellitus – Increased intracranial pressure – Pituitary disorder
Lead	< 150 mcg/24 hour	Increase – Lead poisoning
pH	4.6-8	Increase – Metabolic alkalemia – Proteus infections – Stale specimen
Phenolphthalein (PSP)	25% excreted: 15 min 40% excreted: 30 min 60% excreted: 120 min	Decrease – Congestive heart failure – Renal disease
Protein	0.1 gm/24 hour	Increase – Fever – Infection – Kidney disease – Strenuous exercise
Specific gravity	1.001-1.035	Increase – (Urine more concentrated) – Dehydration Decrease – (Urine less concentrated) – Diuretic therapy – Renal tubular dysfunction
Urea nitrogen	9-16 gm/24 hour	Increase – Excessive protein catabolism

Urine Chemistry (continued)

Constituent	Normal Values	Deviations
Urea nitrogen–(continued)		Decrease – Renal disease
Uric acid	250-750 mg/24 hour	Increase – Gout Decrease – Nephritis

Note: From *Health assessment of the older adult* (pp. 264-271) by C. Eliopoulos, 1984, Menlo Park, CA: Addison-Wesley. Reprinted with permission.

APPENDIX C
RESOURCES

Organizations

Alzheimer's Disease and Related Disorders Association
32 Broadway
New York, NY 10004

American Academy of Geriatric Dentistry
2 N. Riverside Plaza
Chicago, IL 60603

American Art Therapy Association
P.O. Box 11604
Pittsburgh, PA 15228

American Association for Geriatric Psychiatry
230 N. Michigan Avenue, Suite 2400
Chicago, IL 60601

American Association of Homes for the Aging
1050 17th Street, N.W., Suite 770
Washington, D.C. 20036

American Association of Retired Persons
1909 K Street, N.W.
Washington, D.C. 20006

American College of Nursing Home Administrators
4650 East-West Highway
Washington, D.C. 20014

American Foundation for the Blind, Inc.
15 West 16th Street
New York, NY 10011

The American Geriatrics Society
10 Columbus Circle
New York, NY 10019

American Nurses' Association, Inc.
Council of Nursing Home Nurses Division of Gerontological Nursing
2420 Pershing Road
Kansas City, MO 64108

American Psychiatric Association Council on Aging
1700 18th Street, N.W.
Washington, D.C. 20009

American Psychological Association
Division of Adult Development and Aging
1200 17th Street, N.W.
Washington, D.C. 20036

American Public Health Assn. Section of Gerontological Health
1015 18 Street, N.W.
Washington, D.C. 20036

American Speech and Hearing Association
10801 Rockville Pike
Rockville, MD 20852

Commission on Legal Problems of the Elderly
American Bar Association
1800 M street, N.W.
Washington, D.C. 20036

The Gerontological Society of America
1835 K Street, N.W., Suite 305
Washington, D.C. 20006

Gray Panthers
3700 Chestnut Street
Philadelphia, PA 19104

International Center for Social Gerontology
425 13th Street, N.W., Suite 840
Washington, D.C. 20004

The International Federation on Aging
1909 K Street, N.W.
Washington, D.C. 20006

International Senior Citizens Assocation, Inc.
11753 Wilshire Boulevard
Los Angeles, CA 90025

National Action Forum for Older Women
2000 P Street, N.W., Suite 508
Washington, D.C. 20036

National Association of Area Agencies on Aging
1828 L Street, N.W., Suite 404
Washington, D.C. 20036

National Association of Social Workers
1425 H Street, N.W.
Washington, D.C. 20005

National Association of State Units on Aging
1828 L Street, N.W., Suite 505
Washington, D.C. 20036

National Caucus of the Black Aged
1424 K Street, N.W., Suite 500
Washington, D.C. 20005

National Citizens' Coalition for Nursing Home Reform
1424 16th St., N.W., Suite 204
Washington, D.C. 20036

National Council on the Aging
1828 L Street, N.W., Suite 504
Washington, D.C. 20036

National Council of Senior Citizens
1511 K Street, N.W.
Washington, D.C. 20005

National Geriatrics Society
212 W. Wisconsin Avenue
Milwaukee, WI 53203

National Hospice Organization
1331A Dolly Madison Boulevard
McLean, VA 22101

National Interfaith Coalition on Aging
P.O. Box 1904
Athens, GA 30603

National Senior Citizens Law Center
1200 15th Street, N.W.
Washington, D.C. 20005

Journals

Clinical Gerontologist
Hayworth Press
75 Griswold Street
Binghamton, NY 13904

Geriatric Nursing
555 West 57th Street
New York, NY 10019

Geriatrics
7500 Old Oak Boulevard
Cleveland, OH 44130

Geriatrics Survey
Williams and Wilkins
428 East Preston Street
Baltimore, MD 21202

Gerontologist
1411 K Street, N.W., Suite 300
Washington, D.C. 20005

International Journal of Experimental & Clinical Gerontology
S. Karger Publishers
150 Fifth Avenue, Suite 1105
New York, NY 10011

Journal of the American Geriatrics Society
Box 465
Hanover, PA 17331

Journal of Geriatric Psychiatry
64 Hancock Avenue
Newton Centre, MA 02159

Journal of Gerontological Nursing
6900 Grove Road
Thorofare, NJ 08086

Journal of Gerontology
1411 K Street, N.W., Suite 300
Washington, D.C. 20005

INDEX

Page numbers in *italics* indicate figures; page numbers followed by t indicate tables.